The
Natural
Apothecary
Lemons

Other titles in the Natural Apothecary series include:

The Natural Apothecary: Baking Soda
The Natural Apothecary: Cider Vinegar

About the author: Dr Penny Stanway practised for several years as a GP and child-health doctor before becoming increasingly fascinated by researching and writing about healthy diets and other natural approaches to health and wellbeing. Penny has written more than 20 books on health, food and the connections between the two. She lives with her husband on a houseboat in the Thames.

This edition published in the UK and USA 2019 by
Nourish, an imprint of Watkins Media Limited
89–93 Shepperton Road, London N1 3DF
enquiries@nourishbooks.com

3 5 7 9 10 8 6 4 2

Managing Editor: Daniel Hurst
Editor: Amy Christian
Head of Design: Georgina Hewitt
Typeset by: Integra Software Services Pvt. Ltd, Pondicherry
Production: Uzma Taj

Printed and bound in China

A CIP record for this book is available from the British Library

ISBN: 978-1-848993-66-2

Note/Disclaimer: The material contained in this book is set out in good
faith for general guidance and no liability can be accepted for loss or expense
incurred in relying on the information given. In particular this book is not
intended to replace expert medical or psychiatric advice. This book is for
informational purposes only and is for your own personal use and guidance.
It is not intended to diagnose, treat, or act as a substitute for professional
medical advice. The author is not a medical practitioner nor a counsellor,
and professional advice should be sought if desired before embarking on any
health-related programme.

www.nourishbooks.com

DR PENNY
STANWAY

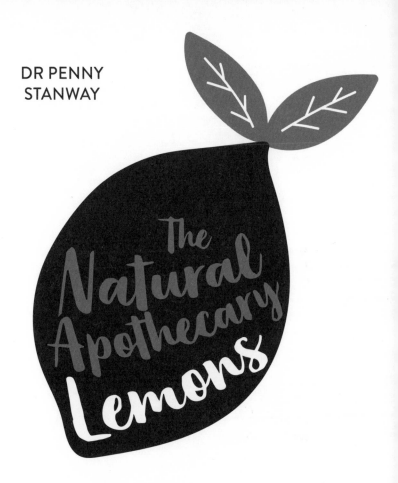

The Natural Apothecary Lemons

USES FOR HOME, HEALTH AND BEAUTY

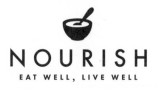

NOURISH
EAT WELL, LIVE WELL

CONTENTS

Introduction   *IX*

Chapter 1   Growing and Buying Lemons   2

Chapter 2   Benefits   12

Chapter 3   Getting the Most from Lemons   38

Chapter 4   Natural Remedies for Health   46

Chapter 5   Natural Beauty Treatments   112

Chapter 6   Natural Cleaning Products   134

Resources   155
Index   156

INTRODUCTION

For many thousands of years, people have been using natural products to soothe, treat, beautify and cleanse. Herbs and spices, vegetables, fruits, nuts and berries (as well as secondary products such as olive oil and vinegar) have been mixed together to create traditional remedies that have been passed down through the generations. Many of these ingredients are still used in commercial products today, although are now often combined with harsh chemicals.

Today, we are used to relying on pharmacies and supermarkets, where there are hundreds of available products, each with a different purpose. We apply creams and ointments for various aches and pains, take vitamin supplements, and spend a fortune on lotions and potions for our skin, nails and hair. The number of cleaning products that are now on offer can be quite overwhelming!

Many fruits are used in natural remedies and homemade products, but the lemon has to be one of the most enduringly popular.

By going back to basics, and taking a more natural approach to how we treat our diets, health, beauty regimes and household management, we are taking back control of what we are putting into our bodies and what we are exposing our families to.

The peel and juice of a lemon has a delightfully fresh citrus aroma and a surprisingly sharp tang, and their wide variety of contents can help us care for our health, beauty and home, and flavour many foods and drinks.

The word 'lemon' comes from the Middle English 'limon', which in turn came from the Old French 'limon', the Italian 'limone', the Arabic 'laymun' or 'limun', the Persian 'limu' and perhaps, originally, the Sanskrit 'nimbuka'.

Lemons are nearly always extremely sour, because they contain a lot of acid but scarcely any sugar. However, this very acidity helps account for their domestic and commercial value, while a little culinary know-how makes them eminently edible and ensures their position among our favourite fruits.

Citrus trees are believed to have originated in central Asia, in the east Himalayan region of India, and Iran. The citrus trees that first came to Europe in the 2nd century were citron trees, which, although very aromatic, contain scarcely any juice. The lemon tree probably resulted from a cross between the citron and the lime, but when and where this happened is unknown.

Lemon trees were well established in Iraq by the end of the 9th century and common in China and the Middle East by the 12th century. The Spanish and Portuguese took lemon seeds from there to Europe in the 15th century, Christopher Columbus took them to Haiti in 1493, and various Spanish adventurers introduced them to the Americas. The Dutch introduced them into South Africa by the middle of the 17th century, and the English took them to Australia in the late 18th century.

Lemons are readily available in grocery stores and supermarkets everywhere, and, lucky for us, are usually inexpensive. For a checklist on what to look out for when selecting lemons, see pages 8–9. If you are green-fingered, lemon trees can be kept outdoors in a warm climate, or in a heated greenhouse or conservatory in a cooler climate (see page 7).

The goodness can be extracted from a lemon in several ways. It can be:

- sliced or in wedges, to get the benefits of the four Ps (peel, pith, pulp and pips)
- zested, using only the bright yellow skin
- juiced (see pages 44–5 for tips on how to get the maximum volume of juice from a lemon)

Every part of a lemon contains beautifying ingredients.

The fruit has many health benefits, and offers a tart and flavourful source of fibre, plus vitamin C and other nutrients. It also provides a wealth of other health-promoting substances (see pages 12–37), some of which occur in such riches in only a few other foods. A surprising number of common ailments can be treated using lemon, see pages 46–111.

Lemon juice can cleanse, soften and moisturize your skin, condition and lighten your hair and deodorize your body. It is often used in commercial beauty products, but similar effects can be achieved at home with inexpensive storecupboard ingredients (see pages 112–133).

Lemons are also useful for many household chores and can help keep your home fresh, clean and sparkling. Note that it is fine to use bottled lemon juice instead of fresh lemon juice for household tasks. For environmentally-friendly, non-toxic ideas for using lemons as a natural cleaning product, see pages 134–155.

INVISIBLE INK

You can amuse children by showing them how to make invisible ink. Simply mix the juice of a lemon with a few drops of water in a small bowl. Then use a cotton bud to write on white paper with this 'ink'. As the ink dries, it should become virtually invisible. To reveal the writing, carefully hold the paper near a light bulb. As the lemon juice heats up, it is oxidized by the air, which darkens it and reveals the writing.

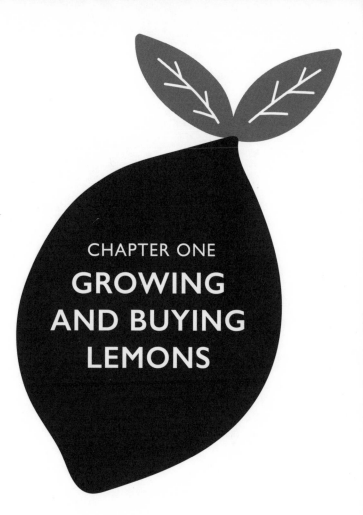

CHAPTER ONE

GROWING AND BUYING LEMONS

I

GROWING AND BUYING LEMONS

The evergreen lemon tree can grow up to 6m/19½ft high. Its fragrant blossoms are white inside, tinged with deep pink outside, and produced all year round. Every other year there is a large total crop of fruit, followed the next year by a lighter one. One tree can produce as many as 500–600 fruits a year (or even, from certain trees, up to 3,000 fruits) in several crops. The peak months for harvesting lemons in the Northern Hemisphere are May, June and August.

The average lemon weighs 75–150g/3–6oz. The lemon is one of the 16 species that make up the Citrus genus. Botanical historians believe that there were originally three species of Citrus tree: *Citrus medica* (the citron), *Citrus maxima* (the pomelo) and *Citrus reticulate* (the mandarin – including the tangerine, satsuma and clementine). The lemon tree (*Citrus limon*), as well as the orange (*Citrus sinensis*), grapefruit (*Citrus paradisi*), Persian lime (*Citrus latifolia*) and key lime (*Citrus aurantifolia*) and other types of citrus tree, originated from the various genetic crosses (hybridizations) of these three original species, or their offspring.

Citrus growers have developed about 47 varieties of lemon tree over many centuries of cultivation. However, lemons come in two main types: those that are relatively more acidic and those that are relatively sweeter. The most widely grown acidic varieties are the Eureka (the sourest lemon, large in size and with thick peel) and the Lisbon (medium-sized, with thin peel and no pips). The more acidic types are mainly grown commercially, whilst sweeter ones are mainly a domestic crop. One of the sweeter types, the Meyer 'lemon', is actually a lemon-mandarin hybrid, so is sweeter, juicier, rounder and less acidic than other lemons and has an orange-yellow colour.

The heaviest recorded lemon in the world was grown in Israel in 2003 and weighed 5.2kg/11½lb).

More than 13 million tonnes of lemons are produced worldwide each year.

Lemon-producing countries include:

- the USA (particularly California and Arizona)
- Mexico
- Argentina
- Chile
- Brazil
- Uruguay
- Spain
- Italy
- Cyprus
- Turkey
- Israel
- Syria
- Iran
- India
- China
- Morocco
- Egypt
- South Africa
- Australia

Growing lemons

Lemon trees grow best in semi-arid and arid subtropical regions of the world, and in temperatures that do not fall below 4°C/39°F. Lemon trees require:

- Warmth and sunshine – outdoors in a warm climate, or indoors in a heated greenhouse or a conservatory in a cooler climate.
- Protection from wind, which can prevent bees pollinating the flowers.
- Excellent drainage, so they should ideally be planted in a clay-free soil on slightly sloping ground.
- Regular feeding with citrus fertilizer (applied at the rate of 120g/4½oz for each year of the tree's age) in January, May and September in the Northern Hemisphere and July, November and March in the Southern. Feed should be spread evenly below the leaf canopy, though not immediately around the trunk.
- Mulching to reduce competition from weeds and to prevent drying out.
- Regular watering, especially in dry weather and during flowering – particularly after pollination.
- Pruning to strengthen shoots, prevent crowding in the centre of the tree, keep the tree to an easily manageable height, and remove diseased and dead wood. Trimming the lower foliage reduces damage from snails and from fungi splashed up from the soil.

NOTE: Pesticide use by commercial growers must adhere to their country's regulations. Domestic growers should take advice from a suitable book or from a nursery or garden centre. The latter two can also advise on the type of lemon

tree that is most suitable for where you live, as trees vary in
the cold tolerance and disease-resistance of their rootstock.

Buying lemons

Ideally, choose lemons that are fresh, healthy and full of
juice. Such a lemon will look good, smell good and taste
good. It will also provide plenty of juice and a firm rind, as
well as nutrients and other health-promoting substances.
When selecting a lemon, check that it:

- Feels firm, full and heavy but has some 'give' when you
  press it – avoid one that is hard and shrivelled (as it be
  may be old and desiccated) or soft and squidgy (as it may
  be decaying).
- Is well shaped and free from scabs or streaks, spots or
  other discoloration, which could be associated with viral,
  bacterial or fungal infection or damage during harvesting
  and post-harvest washing and storage.
- Is free from scars, which could have been caused
  by burning or other injury from pesticide sprays
  or fumigation.
- Is free from pitted or sunken areas on the rind, which
  could have resulted from excessive oil-spraying before
  harvest, or excessive chilling, mechanical brushing or
  humidity afterwards.
- Has bright, shiny yellow peel, which shows it is well
  ripened; a greenish or pale yellow lemon is more acidic.
- Has a uniform colour, which indicates that the peel is
  not infected and the lemon has been well handled.
- Has unbroken peel, since a break could have enabled
  intrusion by infecting micro-organisms.

- Ideally has a coarsely 'pebbled' rind, which indicates that it's likely to keep well.
- Has rough, thick peel if you particularly want its zest, as the yield will be greater.
- Has thin, smooth peel if you particularly want its juice, as the yield will be greater.
- Is unwaxed if you want to use its zest or rind, as it will be free from the wax, fungicide and other substances that are sprayed on lemons during commercial storage. Such lemons are sometimes sold as 'organic'.

When you cut open a lemon, check that it is juicy. Dryness shows that it has been kept too long or is unhealthy. Check too that its pith and membranes are whitish and its pulp pale yellow, since discoloration can be sign of a fungal infection (for example, red, brown or black staining suggests infection with the black-rot fungus, Alternaria, that is most likely to affect trees in wet weather). Discoloration can also result from damage by excessive chilling after a lemon has been harvested.

STORING LEMONS

You can store a lemon for three weeks, perhaps longer, in a sealed plastic bag or a tightly lidded jar in the refrigerator, or for one to two weeks at room temperature and out of direct sunlight.

You can keep lemon juice in an airtight container in the refrigerator for up to five days. Alternatively, you can put juice into ice-cube trays and freeze them for use at a later date.

Lemon zest can be stored in an airtight container in a cool dry place, or put in an airtight freezer bag and frozen. You can also put small strips of lemon zest in water into ice-cube-tray compartments so you can enjoy the look and taste of lemon in ice for drinks.

Lemon slices or wedges (see pages 42–3) can be pre-prepared and kept in a plastic bag in the refrigerator for three or four days.

Added wax, pesticide and other substances

Most lemon farmers spray their trees with pesticides, such as fungicides and insecticides. They may also spray on a growth regulator to make the lemons larger, and spray the ground around the trees with a herbicide to get rid of weeds. Pesticide residues on lemons are washed off in the packing house along with dirt and the lemons' natural wax coating. However, pesticide residues may remain within the lemon's pulp.

Most harvested lemons are sprayed with a water-based emulsion containing wax, a fungicide and, perhaps, a bactericide, a preservative and other substances. The wax helps prevent the loss of moisture and aroma. It also reduces damage during handling, storage and transportation, makes lemons look glossy and accentuates their colour. It may be plant-, insect-, animal- or petroleum-based; carnauba palm wax is the most common. Other compounds sometimes sprayed on after harvesting include ethyl alcohol (to improve the consistency of the wax), casein (to help the wax form an even film) and soap (to aid the flow of the spray).

Unripe green lemons are then stored in climate-controlled conditions for up to 20 weeks, and ripe yellow ones for six weeks. Lemons are sometimes packed in paper wraps, pads or box liners impregnated with diphenyl fungicicide. This is taken up by a lemon's rind but not by its pulp.

The pesticides and herbicides permitted for use on lemons vary from country to country. Many countries test samples of lemons to check that any traces of pesticides and other added chemicals, both on their surface and inside them, are within maximum permitted levels (MPL). If so, the fruit is deemed safe to eat. In the US, pesticide residues are monitored by the Department of Agriculture Pesticide Data Program.

You may prefer to buy organic and unwaxed lemons.

Washing a lemon (see page 41) before consuming it reduces pesticide traces on the peel but not inside the lemon. Depending on each country's regulations, there has generally either been no use of pesticides on lemons allowed to be labelled 'organic', or at least no routine use.

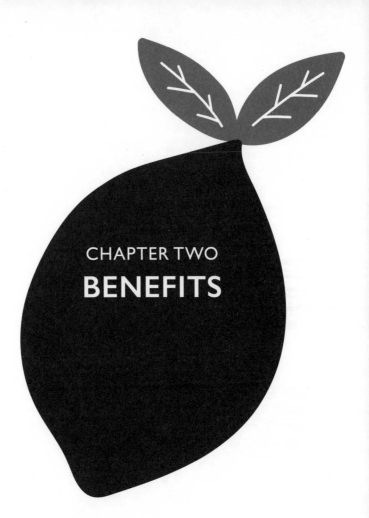

CHAPTER TWO

BENEFITS

BENEFITS

Lemons offer a tart and flavourful source of fibre, plus vitamin C and other nutrients. They also provides a wealth of other health-promoting substances, some of which occur in such riches in only a few other foods, including nutrients, fibre, plant pigments, limonene, organic acids and limonoids.

Nutrients

Lemons are one of the best food sources of vitamin C (an antioxidant also known as ascorbic acid). The antioxidant properties and the acidity of lemons help to explain why they are so beneficial. One small (100g/3½oz) lemon contains 60–100mg of vitamin C. The recommended adult dietary allowance of this vitamin varies between countries, being 90mg a day in the US and 75mg in the UK, for example. So consuming one lemon a day can provide most, if not all, of your daily requirement.

Lemons also contain small amounts of sugar, plant pigments, beta carotene (also called 'pro-vitamin A', as the body makes it into this vitamin), vitamins B and E

It's best to consume lemon juice freshly squeezed, as 20 per cent of its vitamin C is lost after eight hours at room temperature or 24 hours in a refrigerator.

and minerals – particularly potassium, but also magnesium, phosphorus, calcium, copper, iron, manganese, selenium and zinc.

Two-thirds of a lemon's iron is in its peel and pith; two-thirds of its calcium is in its juice. The amounts of vitamins and minerals are small but useful. Lemons also contain minute amounts of proteins and fats, and a medium-sized lemon contains 15 calories of energy.

THE FOUR 'PS'

A lemon has three layers: the peel (which cooks call the zest and botanists call the exocarp, epicarp or flavedo), the pith (mesocarp or albedo) and the pulp (endocarp or flesh). It also has pips, which are in its pulp.

Peel

This is the tough, shiny, textured, vibrant yellow (or green) outer layer. Depending on the variety of lemon and the growing conditions, the peel's thickness varies from a thin 1–2mm/$\frac{1}{16}$–$\frac{1}{8}$ in to a thick 2cm/$\frac{3}{4}$in. Cellulose fibre makes up 30 per cent of the peel. Its other constituents include waxes, organic acids, carotenoid pigments and lemon oil. Tiny oil glands open via pores on to the surface of the peel.

Pith

This is the soft, spongy white lining of the peel. It's mainly composed of fibre but also contains small amounts of antioxidants (such as phenolic compounds and limonin) and other substances.

Pulp

This forms the inside of the lemon and is separated by fibrous membranes into eight to ten segments, each containing tiny ovoid sacs (vesicles) filled with pale yellow juice. This juice forms 20–25 per cent of the weight of a ripe lemon and contains 90 per cent of its vitamin C, as well as small amounts of other antioxidants, plus various vitamins, minerals and organic acids, and lemon oil.

Pips

These are the bitter, whitish seeds in the pulp of most lemons. Their contents include salicylic-acid salts (as in aspirin), limonin and a little lemon oil.

Fibre

A lemon's peel, pith, pips and pulp membranes are rich in valuable dietary fibre (once called 'roughage' but now officially 'non-starch polysaccharides'). Lemons contain two types of fibre: cellulose, which strengthens cell walls, and pectin, which binds cells together.

Cellulose absorbs water in the digestive tract. This makes stools more bulky and less sticky, which helps to prevent constipation and diarrhoea.

Pectin dissolves in the digestive tract to form a gel. Pectin is an antioxidant (see pages 18–21). About 90 per cent of dissolved pectin is fermented by the millions of 'good' bacteria in the bowel, releasing butyric acid and other short-chain fatty acids. These acids are valuable to our health because they:

- Aid the absorption of calcium from the bowel.
- Reduce the absorption of cholesterol from the bowel.
- Suppress the production of cholesterol by the liver while also boosting the proportion of HDL cholesterol (the 'good' type) in the blood.

- Encourage apoptosis ('suicide') of bowel-cancer cells.

Many people don't eat enough fibre. In the US, for example, it has been found that the average intake is only half the recommended amount. Most of us could usefully increase our intake by including suitably prepared lemon peel and pith in recipes for foods and drinks.

Antioxidants

Lemons contain a variety of antioxidants, including many of their phenolic compounds (such as flavonoids and coumarins), as well as vitamins C and E, selenium, zinc, carotenoid pigments, limonin (different from limonene – see pages 23 and 27) and other limonoids, and pectin.

Antioxidants help to protect cholesterol and other body fats from being oxidized by unstable particles known as 'free radicals'. Your body makes more free radicals when it is physically stressed, such as if you smoke too much, expose yourself to too much sun or take too much exercise. The presence of oxidized fats in the body encourages sunburn, prematurely aged skin, infection, pregnancy problems (such as pre-eclampsia and miscarriage), eyesight problems (such as cataracts and age-related macular degeneration), gallstones, high blood pressure, heart attacks, memory loss, strokes and certain cancers. What's more, studies suggest that a lemon's antioxidants enhance the liver's ability to break down toxins by up to 35 per cent.

Many people hope that antioxidant supplements will help protect their health. But these supplements may behave differently to the antioxidants found in lemons and other foods. For example, certain studies show that eating

The good news is that most of us can get all the antioxidants we need from a healthy diet that contains at least five helpings of vegetables and fruit a day – and lemons are an excellent source. vitamin-C-rich fruits and vegetables can reduce the damage to DNA (our cells' genetic material) that can trigger cancer, whilst certain other studies show that using vitamin-C supplements, do not have the same effect.

If you need more antioxidants than usual – for example, in later life, or if you have an infection, feel stressed, or smoke (one cigarette destroys 25mg of the body's vitamin C) – the solution is to eat more antioxidant-rich foods. Including lemons in your diet will give you a great start.

Phenolic compounds

These are present mainly in a lemon's peel and in smaller amounts in its pith and juice. Derived from phenolic acid, and also called polyphenols, their levels vary according to the variety of lemon tree, the maturity of the fruit, the geographical region (because of differing soil chemistry) and the year (because of changing climatic conditions). They include certain flavonoids and coumarins. Many phenolic compounds are antioxidants and some are even more effective than vitamin C.

Flavonoids

These are water-soluble compounds that have also been called citrin, bioflavonoids and vitamin P. The flavonoids in lemons and other citrus fruits are the most biologically active of all the flavonoids in the edible plant kingdom.

The highest concentration is in a lemon's peel and pith. Many lemon flavonoids are antioxidants and some are the yellow pigments that help to give lemon peel its sunny colour. Examples include diosmine, eriocitrin, hesperidin, limotricine, naringin, nobiletin, quercetin and tangeretin. Some of a lemon's antioxidant flavonoids – the polymethoxylated flavones (PMFs) – are dubbed 'super-flavonoids'. The most common are nobiletin and tangeretin. A lemon's peel is 20 times richer than its juice in PMFs. Studies suggest that flavonoids have many health benefits:

- They guard the power of vitamin C by improving its absorption and protecting it from oxidation.
- Super-flavonoids reduce LDL cholesterol (the potentially damaging type) by up to 40 per cent, possibly by reducing its production in the liver.
- Associated with a reduced risk of heart disease.
- They strengthen the walls of our capillaries (tiny blood vessels), so maximizing their potential volume and encouraging good blood flow.
- Their antioxidant power can discourage cancer. For example, naringenin helps to prevent DNA damage and enhances DNA repair.

Hesperidin is one of the most intensively studied antioxidant flavonoids. It can strengthen capillaries, reduce cholesterol and blood pressure, help maintain bone density, discourage infection, have anti-inflammatory and sedative effects, and penetrate the blood–brain barrier (implying it can help to protect the brain from infection or other inflammation). Naringin is a particularly bitter-tasting antioxidant flavonoid, which scientists believe can also help to lower cholesterol.

Another flavonoid, rutin (known in its slightly different form as quercetin), is found in lemon peel and reported to bind ('chelate') potentially harmful heavy metals, so aiding their expulsion from the body.

Coumarins

These are phenolic compounds and their concentrations in a lemon's peel (and mainly in its oil) are up to 100 times higher than in its pulp. They include auraptene, bergamotene, isopimpinellin, limettin, certain psoralens (such as oxypeucedanin, and 5-methoxypsoralen – also known as bergapten), scopoletin and umbelliferone.

Some coumarins can benefit our health because they are antioxidants. For example, studies suggest that auraptene helps prevent degenerative diseases and cancer.

LEMONS AND PHOTOSENSITIVITY

Certain psoralens that are found in lemons (see page 54) can be a problem because they are photoactive. This means that putting lemon oil on the skin makes it extra-sensitive to sunlight. Such photosensitivity can cause either phototoxicity or photo-allergy:

- Phototoxicity produces rapid sunburn that can last for weeks and permanently stain the skin.
- Photo-allergy produces dermatitis (skin inflammation) caused by an immunological reaction transforming a particular skin protein into an antigen ('allergen').

It occurs only in genetically predisposed people who are already sensitized. The rash usually resembles eczema, though there can be uricarial wheals (hives or 'nettle-rash') or hard, thick, itchy patches (lichenoid lesions). The rash can extend to skin that hasn't been in the sun. It resolves if sunlight is avoided.

You can protect yourself from a photosensitive reaction. For example, if you have a massage using a product containing lemon oil, avoid sunlight for 12 hours afterwards. Alternatively, ensure that only one drop of lemon oil in every two teaspoons of carrier oil are used for the massage. And if you zest a lemon, wear rubber gloves or wash your hands afterwards.

Pigments

A lemon's pigments are mainly in its peel. They include carotenoids (orange carotenes, such as beta carotene, and yellow xanthophylls, such as lutein, zeaxanthin, beta cryptoxanthin); green chlorophylls; and yellow flavonoids. As a lemon ripens, it changes from green to yellow as a result of the replacement of chlorophylls with carotenoids.

Lemon pigments promote health. For example:

- High levels of carotenoids in the blood discourage heart disease by helping prevent the oxidation of fats. In particular, they help prevent the oxidation of LDL cholesterol (the potentially damaging sort), and thereby help keep arteries healthy and blood flowing freely.
- Beta carotene and beta cryptoxanthin are converted in the body into vitamin A, which promotes eye health and discourages infection.

Limonin

This and other limonoids (such as nomilin) are antioxidants that belong to a family of substances called terpenoids. Limonin is found throughout a lemon, though mainly in its pith and pips. It is present in about the same amount as vitamin C. Most people say it tastes very bitter. Studies show that limonoids can help prevent cell multiplication in cancers of the mouth, skin, lung, breast, stomach and colon. What's especially interesting is that limonin lasts in the body for up to 24 hours, whereas most other anti-cancer agents in foods remain for much less time. Scientists also suspect that limonin helps prevent the production of LDL cholesterol (the potentially dangerous sort) in the liver.

Organic acids

The acids in lemons include ascorbic acid (vitamin C) (see page 15), citric acid (about 5 per cent of the juice) and glucaric acid. Lemons taste sour because they contain too little sugar to mask their acidity. Most of the acidity is in the juice – and its pH of 2.1 makes this even more acidic than vinegar at pH 2.4–3. (The pH indicates a liquid's acidity or alkalinity: 7 is neutral; below 7 is increasingly acid; above 7 is increasingly alkaline.)

Lemon acids can aid digestion in people who don't make enough of their own gastric acid. After the contents of a lemon or its juice have been digested, the lemon acids are metabolized (broken down) into water and carbon dioxide. The breakdown of the other contents releases alkalizing minerals (calcium, iron, magnesium, potassium, sodium). In contrast, most other fruits (including apples, bananas, grapes, oranges, pears, pineapples) contain so much sugar that their metabolism adds to the body's acid load.

Citric acid

This is an alpha hydroxy acid (AHA), and as such is loved by beauty-product manufacturers for its moisturizing and exfoliating properties (see page 116).

Consuming the citric acid in lemon juice helps move any excess water from the body's tissues into the bloodstream. This reduces congestion in the tissues and enables the blood to flow more freely.

Citric acid is also used in foods and drinks as a preservative and a flavouring (denoted in Europe by the 'E number' E330). It is also put in soaps and laundry detergents (as it makes them foam and work better in hard water), water-softeners, bathroom and kitchen cleaning products, effervescent medications, cosmetics, bath salts and bath 'bombs', and shampoos that remove wax and colouring from hair. It is also used to make concrete set more slowly!

Glucaric acid

This could have important health benefits, as research suggests that it helps to:

- Lower LDL cholesterol (the potentially damaging sort) by up to 35 per cent, but doesn't affect HDL cholesterol (the protective sort).
- Discourage bowel cancer and inflammatory bowel disease by promoting butyric-acid production in the large bowel.
- Prevent oestrogen-sensitive cancer of the breast, prostate, ovary and colon, achieved by suppressing the enzyme

betaglucuronidase. This suppression enables a process called glucuronidation in the liver, which makes oestrogen more water-soluble and so aids its elimination in the urine.

- Prevent pre-menstrual syndrome by encouraging glucuronidation (above).
- Rid the body of pollutants by encouraging glucuronidation (above).

Lemon oil

This pale yellow or green oil, also known as 'lemon essential oil', forms 6 per cent of the weight of a lemon's peel; much smaller amounts are also present in the juice and pips.

It takes around 3,000 lemons to produce 1kg/2lb 4oz of lemon oil.

Enormous volumes of lemon oil are used commercially, for example in soft drinks (such as sodas, lemonades, squashes), foods, soaps, detergents, perfumes and medicines.

Lemon oil has around 300 constituents, including:

- Terpenes – mainly limonene (this forms 90 per cent of the oil; see below), but also citral (5 per cent of the oil; see page 20) and traces of citronellal, farnesenes, geraniol, linalool, myrcene, nerol, nootkatone, pinene, sabinene, terpinene and terpineol.
- Flavonoids, such as diosmin and limotricine.
- Coumarins, such as bergamotene and limettine.
- Hydrocarbons, such as benzanthracene, cymene and sinensal.

- Alcohols, such as nonanol and octanol.
- Aldehydes, such as decanal.
- Methyl anthranilate, which smells strongly of grapes.
- Waxes.

The composition of lemon oil varies according to the type of tree and soil. The extraction method that least alters the oil is cold-pressing, followed by spinning, but the oil may also be:

- Distilled to remove its terpenes; terpene-free oil keeps better and has more aroma as it has a higher concentration of aldehydes.
- Steam-distilled to remove its coumarins and to produce limonene. The resulting oil is psoralen-free, so it can't trigger photosensitive skin reactions.
- Adulterated with synthetic limonene, citral or dipentene.
- Concentrated.
- Treated with preservatives such as BHA (butylated hydroxyanisole) or BHT (butylated hydroxytoluene) to prolong its shelf life.
- Diluted with cheaper oil, such as orange or lime. Orange oil, for example, is ten times cheaper yet contains much the same ingredients, albeit in different percentages (for example, it has much less terpineol).

Lemon oil stimulates the gut and pancreas and, thanks mainly to its limonene content, has antibacterial, antiviral and antifungal properties. It is said to be soothing, relaxing, hypnotic, sedative and anti-inflammatory and also to stimulate the circulation.

When blended with other oils, lemon oil provides a 'top' fragrance note. Its scent is said to lift the spirits, clear the mind and improve concentration. Indeed, the number of typing mistakes halved in a Japanese study in which its vapour was diffused through an office.

Lemon oil should be kept in the dark and used within eight to ten months of opening, since light and air oxidize it, making it cloudy and unpleasant smelling. You can buy lemon oil from various pharmacies and other shops, and online.

Limonene

This (known in a slightly different form as dipentene) is the major component of lemon oil, and a little leaches into the juice. Limonene is a colourless liquid terpene that tastes bitter and smells strongly of oranges. However, its scent is masked by those of other odoriferous compounds in lemon oil – especially by the lilac scent of terpineol (a main fragrance ingredient in lapsang souchong tea, originating from the pine smoke that dried the tea).

Limonene produced by the steam-distillation of lemon oil is used as a flavouring and dietary supplement as well as in fragrances, cosmetic products, medicines and insecticides. It's also a good general-purpose solvent, hence its use in paintstrippers and cleaning products. Our limonene intake depends on our diet. For example, the average daily limonene intake from food in the US as a whole is 16mg but in Arizona it is 70–130mg from citrus fruit alone.

Limonene has important health benefits. For example, it floats on the stomach contents, so if these reflux into the gullet, limonene coats the gullet lining, protecting it from damage by stomach acid. Limonene also speeds stomach emptying, which discourages acid reflux and other causes of indigestion; and it makes a barrier to bacteria that might infect the lining of the stomach and gut.

Limonene also has anti-cancer actions, according to studies that suggest it reduces the incidence and size of certain cancers. In particular, it can:

- Inhibit the cell divisions responsible for stomach, lung, liver and breast cancer; for example, limonene inhibits breast cancer in rats when given pure or as orange oil.
- Encourage a process in the liver called glucuronidation, which aids the elimination from the body of carcinogens and excess oestrogen (associated with oestrogen-dependent cancers of the breast, prostate and bowel).
- Encourage apoptosis ('suicide') of stomach-cancer cells.
- Boost immunity – for example, by encouraging white blood cells to kill cancer cells.

Certain researchers now consider limonene to be a significant anti-cancer agent with potential value as a dietary anti-cancer tool.

Citral
Also known as lemonal, this is the second biggest component of lemon oil. It comprises two terpenoid aldehydes, geranial and neral. These are isomers (meaning virtually identical to each other) and different from two of the other constituents of lemons called geraniol and nerol.

Citral has several possible health benefits. For one thing, it has antimicrobial qualities. For another, studies show that it encourages a process in the liver called glucuronidation – which helps rid the body of unwanted pollutants, hormones and carcinogens.

Lemons and a healthy diet

The easiest way for us to make the most of the goodness that lemons contain is to include them in our daily diet.

The enormous variety of recipes that include lemons emphasizes how useful it is to have lemons available in our kitchen. Most of us are familiar with lemonade, lemon curd and lemon marmalade. We may enjoy lemon and parsley stuffing, candied peel and hollandaise sauce. And we're used to sometimes using lemon juice instead of vinegar in a salad dressing. We can also knock up a soothing drink of hot lemon and honey, and may enjoy lemon-flavoured alcoholic drinks, such as a Margarita, whiskey sour or limoncello.

Many recipes featuring lemons come from Middle Eastern and Mediterranean countries, where lemons are produced and used in abundance.

Avgolemono (egg and lemon soup) and slices of halloumi cheese fried with lemon are two of the best-loved recipes. Pasta coated with lemony, buttery breadcrumbs is a family favourite that is perhaps the ultimate in comfort food and nowadays graces tables far beyond Italy, its mother country.

A squeeze of lemon juice into the cooking pan can lend piquancy to many a vegetable, including green leaves, roots, peas and beans. It's common knowledge that adding lemon juice to cooked fish and shellfish makes them even more delicious, but it's also well worth using lemons when preparing and cooking seafood. For example, lemon juice enhances the flavour of salmon as it cures and of herring as it cooks. Ceviche is a traditional South American dish – a marinade of lemon or lime juice 'cooks' raw fish, making it tender and pale, because the fruit acids break down the long protein molecules.

Lemons also go really well with chicken and other meats, as with a lamb tagine or stuffed cabbage or vine leaves. And you're in for a treat if you slip some halved lemon shells around a sizzling roasting chicken or piece of pork, because heat softens them and mellows their flavour in a most attractive way.

The tartness of lemons and the sweetness of sugar marry exceptionally well, which explains why there are so many popular recipes for lemon-flavoured desserts.

The following recipes are quick and easy ways to add more lemons into your diet. Keep preserved lemons in the storecupboard and add them to soups, stews or tagines. Lemon drinks such as lemonade, lemon barley water and lemon tea are both refreshing and good for you.

Preserved lemons

The distinctive flavour of preserved lemons is essential for a North African tagine (stew). Salting the lemons softens them and drains away any bitterness, while storing them in oil gives them a delightfully mellow flavour.

15 small unwaxed lemons, washed and sliced
3 tbsp sea salt
2 tsp paprika
4 bay leaves
720ml/24fl oz/3 cups walnut or hazelnut oil

1   Layer the lemon slices in a colander, sprinkling each layer with salt. Leave for 24 hours, then pat dry with kitchen paper.
2   Sterilize a 1kg/2lb 4oz well-washed preserving jar by boiling the rubber seal in hot water for 10 minutes, and putting the jar itself into a hot oven for 10 minutes.
3   Lay the lemon slices in the clean jar, sprinkling each layer with a little paprika and inserting a bay leaf every few layers.
4   Cover generously with oil, cover with a disc of waxed paper, then seal and store in a cool dark place. The lemons can be eaten straight away, but will last for 2 years unopened. Once opened, they will keep for 6 months in a refrigerator.

Classic lemonade

Home-made lemonade is always a winner. It's also easy to make, and if you have a blender you can prepare it in hardly any time at all. Drink warm in winter or to soothe a cold, and cold in summer.

3 lemons, sliced and pips
removed
100g/3½oz/scant ½ cup caster
(superfine) sugar

a few ice cubes (optional)

1   With a blender: Put the lemon slices, sugar and 570ml/20fl
     oz/2¼ cups just-boiled water into a blender and whizz until
     smooth. Stir in the same amount of water again.
2   Strain the lemonade into a jug. Drink the lemonade while still
     warm, or let it cool, then add a few ice cubes before serving.
3   Without a blender: Put the lemon slices and sugar into a jug.
     Add 1.1¼0fl oz/4½ cups just-boiled water and stir until the
     sugar has dissolved, pressing the lemons against the side of the
     jug to extract the maximum flavour. Strain the lemonade into a
     jug. Drink the lemonade while still warm, or let it cool and add
     a few ice cubes before serving.

Lemonade variation

This recipe leaves out the lemon pith, making it less bitter than the recipe above.

zest (grated or in strips) and juice of 3 lemons

100g/3½oz/scant ½ cup caster (superfine) sugar
ice cubes

1   Put the lemon zest and juice into a jug, add the sugar and 1.1½ pints/4½ cups just-boiled water and stir until the sugar has dissolved.

2   Strain the lemonade into a jug. Drink the lemonade while still warm, or let it cool and add the ice cubes before serving.

Lemon barley water

This variation of lemonade is not only delicious but is also said to promote health.

75g/3oz/⅓ cup pot (unpearled) barley (barley with its husk and bran removed), washed

3 lemons, chopped
50g/2oz/¼ cup light brown sugar

1   Put the barley and 1.7 ⅓ pints/7 cups just-boiled water in a pan. Bring to the boil, then cover and simmer for 30 minutes.
2   Add the chopped lemons and sugar and leave to cool. Strain the lemonade into a jug and serve. This drink can be kept in a refrigerator for up to 5 days.

LEMON TEA

Simply add a couple of lemon slices or a few wide slivers of lemon zest to a cup or mug of hot black Indian tea, then sweeten the tea with sugar if desired.

Lemon lore

- Note that one medium lemon yields 2–3 tablespoons of juice, 2 teaspoons of grated zest and 7–10 slices.
- Use lemons as soon as possible after cutting them.
- If you have cut a lemon, used part of it and want to store the remainder, either cover the cut surface in clingfilm (plastic wrap) or coat it in vinegar (if it is going to be used in something savoury).
- Brush lemon juice over the cut surfaces of bananas, apples, pears, peaches and avocados that you need to keep for a while, as this keeps their colour by preventing oxidation. Similarly, dip cut white vegetables (such as potatoes or parsnips) in a bowl containing a cupful of water mixed with 1 tablespoon of lemon juice.
- Add a few drops of lemon juice to an electric juicer to help prevent fruit or vegetable juice going brown.
- Add a few drops of juice to cream if it doesn't whip.
- Use a little lemon juice or grated zest instead of salt in recipes, to reduce your intake of sodium.
- Add lemon juice when cooking cauliflower or green vegetables, to brighten their colour.
- Ease peeling of the shells of hard-boiled eggs by adding a squeeze of lemon juice to the water before boiling them.
- When boiling eggs, help prevent their shells cracking by adding a squeeze of lemon juice to the water in the pan.
- When a recipe for cooked food contains lemon juice, add the juice after cooking if possible, as heating increases the loss of vitamin C.
- Add lemon juice when cooking rice, to make it fluffier.
- Intensify the flavour of mushrooms by adding lemon juice when you cook them.

- Add lemon juice when cooking fish, as lemon acids prevent unwanted fishy cooking odours by neutralizing substances called amines in the flesh.
- Make the skin of a roast chicken or duck extra crispy by rubbing it with lemon juice before cooking it.
- Revive a limp lettuce by putting it in a bowl of cold water containing the juice of half a lemon then putting the bowl in the refrigerator for an hour.

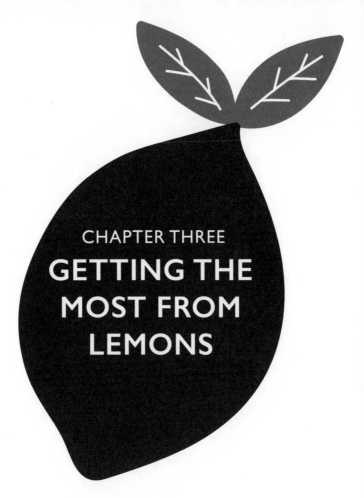

CHAPTER THREE

GETTING THE MOST FROM LEMONS

3

GETTING THE MOST FROM LEMONS

Whether you have grown your lemons, or bought them from a store (see page 8), you will need to wash them. If a lemon is waxed, then before grating or cutting its rind, or before liquidizing it whole, gently brush or rub it with hot water and washing-up liquid for one minute, then rinse it well in plain water.

Most commercially available lemons are sprayed after harvest with an aqueous emulsion of wax (such as carnauba wax) plus a pesticide to prevent them drying out and help avoid infection (see pages 10–11). Alternatively, dip the lemon in just-boiled water for half a minute to dissolve the wax, then remove the lemon and brush it under running water.

The taste of a lemon comes from its acids, its various bitter principles – including limonene (found mainly in a lemon's oil) and limonin, the flavonoid naringin (found mostly in the pith and pips) and its tiny amounts of sugar. The presence of these sour, bitter and sweet substances in saliva is picked up by taste-receptor nerve endings in the taste buds of the tongue and various other parts of the mouth. A few people are genetically unable to detect bitterness in lemons and other foods.

Always remove the zest from a lemon before removing its juice. If you don't need it immediately, you can store it (see page 10) for use later.

After washing the fruit, your method of preparation will depend on how you are planning to use the lemon. Lemons are best cut into wedges or slices so that you can easily get to the zest or juice, as required.

Lemon wedges

There are several ways to prepare lemon wedges ('quarters') to accompany fish or other dishes so the user won't get sprayed with juice when squeezing the juice from the wedge. First, cut the lemon in half lengthways, then cut each half into two or three wedges, depending on the size of the lemon. Next, choose one of the following:

- Best of all, cut a tiny piece from the two pointed ends of the wedge with a sharp knife, then use sharp scissors to cut off any of the lemon's central white core, and to dig out the pips.
- Wrap the wedge in a circle of muslin, secured by knotting its free edges or binding them with fine string; while this looks wonderful, you may think it over the top.
- Give each diner a little hinged lemon press (available from cook shops).

Lemon slices

To prepare lemon slices, cut the lemon in half crossways, then cut slices crossways from each half.

To prepare notched-edge slices, take a lemon slice and cut notches in its peel.

To prepare lemon twists as a garnish for food or drinks, take a lemon slice, cut it from its centre to its edge, then twist each cut end in opposite directions. Secure with a cocktail stick if using for a drink.

Be wary of accepting lemon slices in drinks in restaurants and pubs, since they could make you unwell unless prepared with scrupulous hygiene. The background to this is a study in New Jersey in which researchers ordered drinks containing lemon slices at 21 restaurants. Tests showed that 77 per cent of the lemon slices contained staphylococci, Shigella (dysentery bacteria), or other infectious organisms. This probably means that the restaurant employees either handled the lemons without first washing their hands with anti-bacterial soap (a severe violation of the health code in most US states), or that they cut raw meat, then used the unwashed knife to cut the lemons.

Lemon zest

There are various ways to remove the zest, depending on the result you want:

- For finely grated zest, use a metal grater, taking care to move the lemon frequently, and not to grate your fingers! (Use a stiff pastry brush to remove the zest from the grater.)

- For very fine 'julienne' strips, use a citrus zester.
- For wider strips, use a vegetable paring knife or a vegetable peeler, cutting the zest either down the length of the lemon or in one continuous spiral strip around the lemon; cut the strips with a sharp knife to make them thinner, if necessary.
- For yellow-stained zesty sugar, rub the zest off with sugar lumps, then use them in recipes.

> When grating zest for decoration, grate only the yellow part, not the white pith beneath too, as this is particularly bitter. However, when producing zest to include in a healthy diet, or for medicinal reasons, it's fine to include some grated pith, as its flavonoids and other phenolic compounds are good for us.

Lemon juice

To get the maximum volume of juice from a lemon, it needs to be at room temperature. If it has been kept in a fridge, remove it a couple of hours before juicing it. Alternatively, put it in a bowl and cover with just-boiled water for half a minute. Next, roll the lemon with your hand on a flat surface, as this helps to release the juice by breaking down the lemon's internal membranes. Finally, squeeze out the juice using one of the following:

- Your hands.
- A citrus reamer (a plastic, wooden, metal or ceramic ribbed rounded-cone-shaped device that you twist into the lemon).

- A citrus trumpet (a metal gadget that you screw into the lemon, then squeeze the lemon juice by hand into it).
- A lemon squeezer (a glass, ceramic or metal ribbed device with a pip catcher and a juice-collecting area).
- An electric lemon squeezer.

You can add the leftover lemon pulp to the juice if you want.

BOTTLED LEMON JUICE

Lemon juice is available to buy in a bottle. This can be handy if you get caught short, but it does not taste nearly as good as fresh juice. One reason is that the contents of bottled juice are slightly different from those of fresh juice: for example, there is less vitamin C in bottled juice. Another reason is that it's likely to contain preservatives, such as sodium benzoate or sodium metabisulfite. (It's worth noting here that sodium metabisulfite can trigger an allergic reaction in certain people.) On the plus side, though, bottled juice is usually cheaper than fresh juice, and it also lasts longer, so you may like to use it in home-made cleaning products (see Chapter 6).

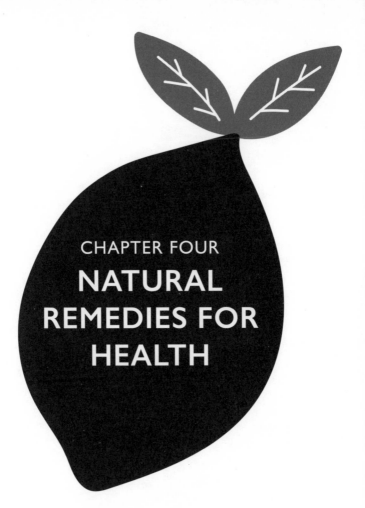

CHAPTER FOUR
NATURAL REMEDIES FOR HEALTH

4

NATURAL REMEDIES FOR HEALTH

Lemons have long been prized as an aid to health. Their health-giving components include antiseptics, antifungals, antivirals, diuretics, astringents, tonics, antioxidants, detoxifiers, anticancer agents, anti-inflammatories and antihistamines.

Traditional use, common sense and anecdotal evidence suggest that lemons can help many different ailments, but few scientific trials have been done because funding is problematic as lemons and their components cannot be patented.

Many people are now choosing to start their day with a cup of hot water and lemon, rather than reaching for the tea or coffee. This is said to aid digestion and kick-start the metabolism, as well as giving the body a boost of vitamin C.

The list of ailments in this chapter details how and why lemons can help, but don't forget that you can also discourage common ailments with a healthy diet, adequate hydration, regular exercise, daily outdoor light, effective stress management, a sensible alcohol intake and no smoking.

PLEASE NOTE

- The strategies outlined should not take the place of medical diagnosis and therapy.
- Avoid lemons if you are allergic to them.
- The acidity in lemons may temporarily soften tooth enamel, making it vulnerable to damage, so dilute their juice and either use a straw to consume drinks containing lemon juice or rinse your mouth with water afterwards.
- Don't brush your teeth soon after you have finished a lemon drink, as this might cause micro-abrasions of your softened tooth enamel.

When including lemon juice and zest in your diet, remember that you can take them in water, lemonade (see pages 32–3) or a wide variety of foods, including salad dressings, sauces, salsas, soups, casseroles, grills, cakes, breads and pies. You can also cook lemon slices with fish and roast the empty 'shells' of squeezed lemons with vegetables or meat, as cooking softens the rind.

Skin and hair

Acne
One possible cause is over-production of sebum caused by oversensitivity of sebaceous glands to testosterone. Others include changes in sebum, and unusually sticky hair-follicle cells. Triggers include the pre-menstrual fall in

oestrogen, humidity, stress, certain drugs (for example, the progestogen-only Pill) and polycystic ovary syndrome. A reduction in the skin's acidity may encourage infection with acne bacteria. Lemon juice may help because it kills acne bacteria, increases skin acidity, 'cuts' (emulsifies) skin oil and reduces inflammation.

Regular treatment
Apply lemon juice with a cotton pad 2 or 3 times a day.

Age spots
The most common are brown age freckles caused by normal ageing plus photo-ageing (accelerated ageing from sun exposure). Some people say lemon juice lightens age spots.

Regular treatment
Apply lemon juice to the affected area each day, and the spots may begin to lighten within 6 weeks.

Heal from the inside out
Include the zest and juice of a lemon in your daily diet, as their antioxidants may delay age freckles and other signs of ageing of the skin.

Chapped lips
Lemon juice can be soothing when the skin on the lips is dry and peeling (especially common in cold temperatures).

Quick fix
Stir a few drops of lemon juice into half a teaspoonful of Vaseline (petroleum jelly) or glycerine and smooth over your lips.

Chilblains
Lemon flavonoids can help the swelling and itching by reducing leakage of fluid from your capillaries (tiny blood vessels) into your skin.

Heal from the inside out
Include the juice and zest of a lemon in your daily diet.

Corns and calluses
Ill-fitting footwear is usually to blame. Soaking the hard skin regularly in lemon juice and water, or lemon essential oil, should soften and hasten its replacement with healthy skin.

Regular treatment
Add the juice of two lemons to a basin of warm water and soak your feet for 10 minutes a day. Then rub the softened skin away.

Intensive foot treatment for hard skin

This works best if the treatment is repeated every day for one week.

1 drop lemon oil

2 teaspoons sweet almond oil
(or other carrier oil)

1   Mix the lemon oil with the sweet almond oil in a small bowl.
2   Massage the oil into hard skin areas on your feet with your
    fingers, making sure to rub it in well.
3   Wrap your foot or feet in clingfilm (plastic wrap), and sit back
    and relax for 20 minutes.
4   Remove the clingfilm (plastic wrap) and dry your feet off with
    a towel.

Itching
Lemon juice is said to reduce itching.

Regular treatment
Bathe in tepid bath water containing the juice of 2 lemons.

Quick fix
Apply lemon juice directly to itchy skin.

Warts
Both lemon juice and lemon oil are reputed to help cure warts.

Heal from the inside out
Consume the juice of half a lemon twice a day at least.

Regular treatment
Apply 1 drop of lemon essential oil to your wart and cover with a sticking plaster. Repeat each day for 2 weeks.

Psoriasis
Patches of thick flaking skin overlie inflammation on the knees, elbows, scalp or elsewhere. Citric acid in lemon juice can ease dryness and flaking. In addition, the sun's ultraviolet-A rays act on psoralens in lemon juice to mimic the PUVA (psoralen-UVA) therapy used for psoriasis by dermatologists. The anti-inflammatory effects of a lemon's carotenoids and certain flavonoids (such as hesperidin) may soothe inflammation.

Regular treatment
Smooth lemon juice over psoriasis several times a day. Treat patches with juice, as above, then expose them to sunlight for a few minutes a day, increasing the time over several weeks.

Heal from the inside out
Include the zest and juice of a lemon in your daily diet.

Dandruff
This flakiness is often associated with infection with the fungus Malassezia furfur. Lemon juice or oil may help.

Regular treatment
Apply a cup of lemon juice to the scalp, cover with a towel for 1 hour, then rinse and shampoo. Repeat once or twice a week.

Anti-dandruff treatment for dry scalps

2 teaspoons coconut oil

1 drop lemon essential oil

1 drop chamomile essential oil

1   Warm the coconut oil in a small pan over a low heat. When liquid, pour the melted oil into a bowl.
2   Add the drops of essential oil and mix well.
3   Massage the mixture into your scalp for 5 minutes.
4   Cover your hair and scalp with a hot towel for 20 minutes.
5   Wash hair with a mild shampoo to remove the treatment.

Head lice

Lemon oil has been shown to deter head lice.

Quick fix

Add 2 drops of lemon oil to your shampoo, and also add 2 drops to your conditioner or final rinse.

Digestion, diet and gut health

Anaemia

Iron-deficiency anaemia can be associated with low levels of stomach acid. This reduces iron absorption from food; it can also be associated with vitamin B12-deficiency anaemia.

Low stomach acid affects one in two over-60s and can result from ageing, stress, the prolonged use of acid-suppressant medication, and an unhealthy diet high in meat, grain, sugar and carbonated drinks (which produce acid in the body) but low in vegetables and fruits.

In someone who lacks stomach acid, a lemon's acidity could aid digestion by lowering the pH of the stomach.

Some alternative practitioners suggest, though without proof, that sodium from fruits and vegetables could help prevent the body diverting sodium from stomach-acid-producing cells and thus reducing stomach acid. They say this frees sodium to 'partner' acids in the urine and thereby remove excess acidity from the body.

In addition, a lemon's pectin is broken down by gut bacteria, releasing short-chain fatty acids, which boost iron absorption by raising acidity.

Heal from the inside out
Drink a glass of water containing 2 teaspoons of lemon juice before each meal.

Constipation
An unhealthy diet and dehydration are the likeliest causes of constipation. Lemons are mildly laxative, partly because they are rich in pectin. This dissolves to form a gel in the bowel that makes stools softer and easier to pass. The cellulose in lemons also attracts water. This makes stools bulkier, softer and easier to pass, and reduces their transit time.

Heal from the inside out
Include the zest and juice of a lemon in your daily diet.

Diarrhoea
Lemons might help in several ways. Their pectin dissolves in the gut to form a gel. This helps bind the bowel contents into stools, which increases transit time. Also, 'good' gut bacteria break down some of the pectin. This forms a coating for the gut lining, which soothes irritation. It also releases butyric acid and other short-chain fatty acids with prebiotic qualities, meaning they nourish good ('probiotic') bowel bacteria such as lactobacilli and bifidobacteria. All this helps colon cells produce mucus, which helps prevent irritants sticking to and inflaming the gut lining. The cellulose in lemons attracts water in the bowel, making its contents more bulky and less runny. Food acid, like stomach acid, helps kill diarrhoea-causing bacteria such as Escherichia coli.

Lemons are particularly useful for people (such as one in two over-60s) with poor stomach-acid production. Indeed, certain West African villagers consume citric acid with a meal to protect themselves from cholera. The acidity of lemons (pH 2.1) is only a little less than that of stomach acid (pH 1–2). The hesperidin that's concentrated in lemon pith may reduce bowel inflammation.

Heal from the inside out
Include the zest and juice of a lemon in your daily diet.

Gallstones

Most gallstones contain cholesterol; others contain bile pigments or calcium salts. Cholesterol-laden bile, and a poorly contracting gallbladder that can't expel small stones, are encouraged by obesity, constipation and diabetes. Bile can become unhealthily acidic, for example in people who eat an unhealthy diet, and stones are more likely to form in acidic bile. A lemon's pectin helps bind bile acids in the gut, which prevents them from being reabsorbed and used to make gallstones.

Acidic foods such as lemon juice encourage the gallbladder to contract and expel bile and small stones. A lack of stomach acid (as with ageing, stress, and medication with antacids or acid-suppressants) discourages gallbladder contractions, and stones readily form in stagnant bile. Lemon juice before a meal can mimic stomach acid. Lemons as part of a healthy diet discourage any tendency of the body to become relatively more acidic. Lemons may also discourage acidity and gallstones, and certain practitioners suggest, though their suggestions are unproven, that their sodium may encourage the production of stomach acid.

GALLBLADDER FLUSH

Consult with your doctor before trying this.

Days 1–6:   Drink 1 litre/35fl oz/4 cups of apple juice a
day for 6 days.

Day 7:   The next day, miss supper.
At 9pm, take 1–2 tablespoons of Epsom salts
in a little water.
At 10pm, drink 4 tablespoons of lemon juice
shaken with 125ml/4fl oz/½ cup of olive
oil, then lie on your left side for 30 minutes
before bedtime.

A 'gallbladder flush' aims to soften stones and encourage gallbladder contractions and may be worth trying. Studies suggest that antioxidants discourage gallstones.

Heal from the inside out
Include the zest and juice of 2 lemons in your daily diet.

Regular treatment
If you have stones, take 1 tablespoon each of lemon juice and olive oil 1 hour before breakfast each day.

Indigestion and heartburn
Lemon juice makes fried food more digestible because its acids emulsify ('cut') fats, so that they don't lie on the stomach, and aid protein digestion – which is particularly useful for the many people who lack sufficient stomach acid, such as one in two over-60s, and those who are stressed or

take antacids unnecessarily. Also, lemons are metabolized to potassium carbonate, which helps reduce any excess acidity in the body. Finally, limonene may help prevent heartburn (perhaps by coating the gullet lining and thus protecting it from acid) and promote healthy stomach movements.

Heal from the inside out
Include the zest and juice of a lemon in your daily diet.

Quick fix
Drink 1 tablespoon of juice in a glass of warm water.

Irritable bowel syndrome (IBS)
Possible symptoms include pain, constipation, diarrhoea, passing mucus, bowels never feeling empty, wind and bloating. One in three people sometimes has an irritable bowel; one in five of these has frequent trouble, known as irritable bowel syndrome. The pectin in lemons may reduce symptoms by making stools softer and easier to pass.

Heal from the inside out
Include the zest and juice of a lemon in your daily diet.

Food intolerance
This can be associated with a lack of stomach acid (such as with stress, ageing, the unnecessary use of antacids or an unhealthy, acid-producing diet high in meat, grain, sugar and carbonated drinks but low in organic sodium from vegetables and fruits). Stomach acid enables the digestive enzyme pepsin to break down proteins; a shortage allows fragments of poorly digested protein to be absorbed into the blood, where they may trigger allergy.

A lemon's acids can mimic the action of stomach acid. Some practitioners say, though without proof, that the sodium in fruits and vegetables can help the body deal with an acidproducing diet by 'partnering' acids so they can escape in the urine. They say this means the body does not have to divert sodium from stomach-acid producing cells, which would prevent the proper production of stomach acid.

Heal from the inside out
If you suspect you lack stomach acid, start each main meal with a salad dressed with lemon juice and olive oil, or a glass of water containing 2 teaspoons of lemon juice.

Kidney stones
Lemons can help prevent stones by providing calcium, magnesium, selenium, vitamin B and fibre.

In particular, consuming lemon juice may help dissolve stones that contain uric acid or calcium. Calcium-containing stones are more likely to form when threatened over-acidity of body fluids leads to calcium being withdrawn from bones and teeth and excreted in the urine to help keep the pH (acid–alkaline balance) of body fluids within its normal range.

The metabolism of the acids in lemon juice has a mild alkalinizing effect in the body, so consuming lemon juice could help prevent this type of stone.

Stones are also more likely in people with pre-diabetes, as their raised blood sugar level after eating carbohydrate raises insulin, which, in turn, makes their kidneys discharge calcium in the urine. A lemon's acidity discourages high blood sugar.

Heal from the inside out
Include the zest and juice of a lemon in your daily diet.

Quick fix

To reduce pain from a stone, drink the juice of half a lemon in a glass of water every half an hour for 4 hours or until the pain subsides.

Peptic ulcer

An ulcer can develop if something interferes with the stomach's protective mucus, lining cells or acid. Unfortunately, many people lack stomach acid, including one in two over-60s and many of those who are stressed, are habituated to antacids or acid suppressants, or eat an acid-producing diet rich in meat, grain, sugars and carbonated drinks and low in fruits and vegetables. Inflammation from infection with Helicobacter pylori bacteria is a major cause of stomach ulcers, inflammation (gastritis) and cancer. Around two in five of us are infected, though only one in 10 infected people get an ulcer. It's a common misconception that people with ulcers make too much acid. In fact, most don't, and many make too little.

Japanese research has indicated a strong correlation between low stomach acidity and increased rates of H. pylori infection. It's possible that if someone with peptic ulcer symptoms tests positive for H. pylori and suspects a lack of stomach acid (for example, because antacids don't relieve their symptoms), the acidity of lemon juice might discourage the infection.

Also, a lemon's sodium can help the body deal with an acid-producing diet by 'partnering' acids so that they can escape in the urine. This means the body does not have to divert sodium from stomach-acid producing cells to do this. This is good, because sodium is necessary for stomach-acid production.

Heal from the inside out
Drink a glass of water containing 2 teaspoons of lemon juice with each meal, or add lemon juice to some of your everyday recipes.

Obesity

Lemons contain pectin, which forms a gel in the digestive tract. This mops up triglyceride fats and reduces their absorption; it also increases satiety. Lemon acids and pectin slow the absorption of sugar after a meal with a high glycaemic index (blood-sugar-raising effect), which in turn slows the rise in blood sugar. This helps prevent low blood-sugar dips, which can trigger overeating.

If the stomach produces too little stomach acid, calcium is absorbed in an insoluble form, which means it cannot be ionized and absorbed in the bowel. The sodium in fruits and vegetables may help prevent a lack of stomach acid due to an acid-producing diet. This is because it can 'partner' acids so that they can escape in the urine. This means that the body does not have to divert sodium from stomach-acid-producing cells. This is good news because sodium is vital for the production of stomach acid.

The vitamin C in lemons could aid weight loss, too. We need adequate vitamin C to produce enough carnitine – an amino acid that helps our body burn fat well.

Heal from the inside out
Include the zest and juice of a lemon in your daily diet.

Circulation issues

Ankle swelling
The flavonoid rutin in lemons strengthens vein walls, so may reduce ankle swelling caused by fluid seeping from varicose veins. Lemons may also ease any fluid retention associated with heart or kidney disease because they have diuretic action – meaning they increase urine production.

Heal from the inside out
Include the zest and juice of a lemon in your daily diet.

Cellulite
This dimpling of the skin is associated with excess tissue fluid and, perhaps, with unhealthy, inelastic collagen fibres tethering the skin. Lemons can act as a diuretic, helping expel excess tissue fluid. They are also rich in vitamin C, which is needed for healthy collagen.

Heal from the inside out
Include the zest and juice of a lemon in your daily diet.

Circulation-boosting bath

The combination of the oils with a brisk massage will boost circulation in affected areas.

2 drops lemon oil   2 drops cypress oil

1   Run a warm bath, and add the lemon and cypress oils.
2   While bathing, massage your skin with a loofah.

Mental health

Anxiety
Eating lemons might reduce anxiety or even panic attacks. Researchers have found that the urine of people with panic attacks is unusually acidic. Unusually acidic urine suggests that the kidneys are trying to prevent threatened over-acidity of the body. One reason could be an unbalanced diet with a lot of grain, sugar and meat but insufficient vegetables and fruit. Lemons can help the body maintain its normal pH (acid–alkaline balance).

Heal from the inside out
Consume the juice of one or two lemons each day.

Depression
The scent of lemon oil can affect mood, possibly via the brain's limbic system. Researchers have found that inhaling lemon-oil vapour can ease a depressed mood.

Regular treatment
Put a few drops of lemon essential oil into a diffuser or on a paper tissue and inhale the vapour every so often.

Stress
The body's need for certain nutrients – including vitamins B and C, calcium, magnesium, potassium and zinc – rises during stress. Lemons can help with their supply. In addition, the scent of lemon oil is said to alleviate stress.

Heal from the inside out
Include the zest and juice of a lemon in your daily diet.

Quick fix
Consider using a few drops of lemon essential oil in an aromatherapy diffuser or massage blend.

Age-related conditions

Ageing

Elderly people absorb less nourishment, which can
contribute to premature ageing. Indeed, a recent UK survey
noted that one in ten over-65s were short of iron and
vitamins B and C, all of which lemons can help provide.
Studies suggest that antioxidants discourage premature
ageing of the skin. Vitamin C and other antioxidants in
lemons might help counter premature ageing elsewhere in
the body, too – for example, in joints and blood vessels.
What's more, in Westernized cultures lemon acids could
help the one in two over-60s who have an agerelated
reduction in stomach acid, because this makes many of
them unable to absorb certain nutrients properly. US
researchers have found that certain mineral and vitamin
deficiencies accelerate age-related decay of mitochondria
(the energy-providing structures in cells).

Scientists have long searched for lifestyle factors that
encourage long life and discourage age-related diseases such
as arthritis, heart disease, diabetes, cancer, osteoporosis and
Alzheimer's.

Long-lived peoples include certain groups in Russia,
Pakistan, Ecuador, China, Tibet and Peru. One link is
that many live at high altitudes, where glacier water is rich
in alkaline minerals such as calcium. Such minerals help
the body maintain a healthy pH (acid–alkaline balance)
without drawing calcium from the bones. Lemon juice can
have a similar effect.

Another factor linking many of these long-lived peoples
is their consumption of lactic and acetic acids from
fermented vegetables, fruit, milk, cereal grain, sugars, meat

and fish. Like lemon acids, these help the body maintain a healthy pH.

Consuming vinegar before a meal discourages high blood sugar afterwards. Experts say the acids in lemon juice mean it's likely to behave in the same way.

The antioxidants in lemons may also reduce the inflammation associated with heart disease, arthritis and Alzheimer's (see page 69).

Lemon consumption may also discourage certain cancers, and strokes. It's said that the vitamin C a person gets by consuming lemon juice each day can raise their life expectancy by 6 years.

Finally, pectin encourages the elimination of toxic heavy metals, such as aluminium and lead, in the gut (and is prescribed for this purpose in Russia). Such metals encourage premature degeneration and ageing of brain and other cells. A lemon's peel, pith and segment walls are rich in pectin.

Heal from the inside out
Include the zest and juice of a lemon in your daily diet.

Cataracts
Clouding of the eye's lens affects many over-65s. Risk factors include diabetes, high blood pressure, smoking, infection and sunlight. Studies suggest that the antioxidant power of vitamin C lowers the risk of cataracts by 80 per cent. Lemons are rich in antioxidants.

Heal from the inside out
Include the zest and juice of a lemon in your daily diet.

Macular degeneration

Vitamin C in food discourages age-related macular degeneration (AMD, deterioration of 'straight-ahead' sight), say Dutch researchers. They followed up 4,170 over-55s for about eight years, and found that the 560 who developed AMD ate less vitamin-C-rich food than the others. Supplements of vitamin C made no difference.

Heal from the inside out

Include the zest and juice of a lemon in your daily diet.

Arthritis

Inflammation links most kinds of arthritis. Lemon antioxidants help reduce inflammation. Some people believe they should avoid lemons because they are acidic. But we metabolize lemon acids to potassium carbonate, which helps prevent excess acidity in our body.

Hesperidin, concentrated in lemon pith, is an anti-inflammatory antioxidant, so may reduce joint inflammation.

A 2004 study of more than 20,000 subjects who kept diet diaries and were arthritis-free when the study began, indicates that vitamin C rich foods such as lemons can help protect against inflammatory polyarthritis, a form of rheumatoid arthritis involving two or more joints. This arthritis was more than three times as likely in those who consumed the least vitamin C-rich food as in those who ate the most.

Heal from the inside out

Include the zest and juice of a lemon in your daily diet.

Soothing massage oil

1 drop lemon oil

1 drop pine oil

2 teaspoons sweet almond oil
(or other carrier oil)

1   Mix together the lemon and pine oils with the sweet almond oil in a small bowl.
2   Gently massage the oil mixture into the joints.

Memory loss

Lemons are rich in antioxidants, and studies of mice suggest these discourage memory loss.

Heal from the inside out

Include the zest and juice of a lemon in your daily diet.

Osteoporosis

Affected bone is light and fragile. Risk factors include a lack of 'bone-friendly' nutrients, such as calcium, magnesium, zinc and vitamin C. Lemons help provide these. Researchers suspect that inflammation may play a part in osteoporosis; lemons provide anti-inflammatories such as nobiletin. Other risk factors for osteoporosis include age, too much exercise and smoking. These encourage oxidation by free radicals, which research increasingly suggests may be an underlying factor. Lemons contain a wide variety of antioxidants.

Lemon pectin may be useful, too, because gut bacteria break it down, releasing short-chain fatty acids (such as butyric acid), which raise acidity in the large bowel. This boosts the absorption of bone-friendly minerals such as calcium and magnesium.

Lemons as part of a healthy diet help prevent any tendency of the blood to be at the lower (and hence relatively more acidic) end of the normal range of pH (acid–alkaline balance – the normal range being 7.35–7.45). This is because lemons are metabolized in the body to produce alkaline end-products. This helps prevent the need for the body to take calcium and other minerals from the bones in order to accompany and thus get rid of acid in the urine. A diet rich in meat, grain, sugars and carbonated soft drinks encourages a tendency to increased acidity in the blood; a diet rich in vegetables and fruits such as lemons discourages it.

Finally, lemon acids provide acidity in the stomach for those who lack enough for good calcium absorption. A lack of stomach acid can reduce calcium absorption by 80 per cent. It affects one in two over-60s and is more common in people who are stressed, habitually take antacids or acid-suppressants, or eat an acid-producing diet high in meat, grain, sugar and carbonated drinks and low in fruit and vegetables. A lemon's sodium can help the body deal with such a diet by 'partnering' acids so that they can escape in the urine. This means the body does not have to divert sodium from stomach-acid producing cells, and in so doing prevent the proper production of stomach acid.

Heal from the inside out
Include the zest and juice of a lemon in your daily diet.

Alzheimer's disease
This condition destroys brain cells and is associated with patches of amyloid protein and clusters of tangled nerve fibres in the brain. Experts believe that inflammation is partly to blame. Also, research suggests that damage from oxidation of the brain's two most abundant polyunsaturated fatty acids – docosahexaenoic acid and arachidonic acid – contributes to Alzheimer's. Finally, affected people have high levels of the amino acid homocysteine. A lack of B vitamins raises homocysteine levels, and sufferers are particularly likely to go short of these vitamins. Lemons may help, as they contain antioxidants, other anti-inflammatories and B vitamins.

Laboratory tests in the US and Korea reveal that the antioxidant quercetin helps protect rat brain cells from oxidation.

Lemons contain anti-inflammatories such as hesperidin, which can penetrate the blood–brain barrier.

Heal from the inside out
Include the zest and juice of a lemon in your daily diet.

Respiratory problems and allergies

Hay fever
Lemons might discourage hay fever and other allergic rhinitis because they contain anti-inflammatories and antihistamines, which may help prevent or ease an attack.

Heal from the inside out
Include the zest and juice of a lemon in your daily diet.

Regular treatment
During an attack, consume 2 tablespoons of lemon juice in a glass of water three times a day.

Quick fix
If your throat is sore, gargle with 1 tablespoon of lemon juice in a cup of warm water.

Asthma
Inflammation and oversensitivity of the airways causes wheezing, a cough and tightness of the chest. Triggers include cold air, exercise, certain foods, hormone changes, laughter, infection, fumes, suddenly reduced air-pressure, thunderstorms, allergy and rapid breathing.

Lemons contain anti-inflammatory antioxidants. One of these, quercetin, also acts as an antihistamine.

In 1931, Dr George W. Bray of The Hospital for Sick Children, London, measured stomach acid after a meal in more than 200 children with asthma. Astonishingly, 9 per cent had none, 48 per cent had a severe lack and 23 per cent had a slight lack. So four in five lacked sufficient stomach acid! Other researchers have found a lack of stomach acid in many adults with asthma. One possible cause of allergic sensitization of the lining of the airways is absorption from the gut into the blood of poorly digested protein particles – which can be associated with low stomach acid. This is extraordinarily interesting but largely ignored. It's possible for low stomach acid to be encouraged by an acid-producing diet rich in grain, sugars, meat, dairy and carbonated drinks and low in fruit and vegetables. Some alternative practitioners suggest, though without proof, that a deficiency of sodium from fruits and vegetables encourages the body to remove sodium from various places – including stomach-acid-producing cells – so it's available to escort acid from the body in the urine. They say this could reduce stomach acid production.

Regular treatment
If you suspect that you have low stomach acid (for example, because you get indigestion unrelieved by antacids), try taking 2 teaspoons of lemon juice three times a day to help prevent asthma.

Quick fix
Alternatively, take lemon juice early in an attack. For an adult, put 1 tablespoon of lemon juice in a glass of water and sip it over half an hour. Wait for half an hour, then repeat. For a child, use less, depending on their size. Asthma medication prescribed by a doctor should also be taken.

First aid and infections

Bites and stings
Wasp stings irritate because they are alkaline, so lemon acids may help. They may also ease irritation from mosquito and gnat bites.

Quick fix
For a wasp sting or mosquito or gnat bites, apply a cotton pad soaked in lemon juice, and repeat if necessary.

Bruises
These result from damage that makes blood leak from tiny blood vessels. Lemon peel and juice may limit bruising and speed recovery because their flavonoids strengthen blood-vessel walls.

Heal from the inside out
Include the zest and juice of a lemon in your daily diet.

Cuts and grazes
A lemon's antiseptic properties can be useful for dealing with minor cuts and grazes.

Quick fix
Gently clean the skin with a cotton pad soaked in lemon juice.

Nosebleed
Lemon juice has astringent properties, and a lemon's peel, pith and core are rich in rutin and other flavonoids that can strengthen blood vessels.

Quick fix
Soak a cotton ball in lemon juice, lean your head backwards, then put the ball in the affected nostril and leave for 10 minutes.

Heal from the inside out
If you have frequent nosebleeds, include the zest and juice of a lemon in your daily diet.

Fishbone in throat
Lemon acids could soften a small fishbone and encourage it to be dislodged.

Quick fix
Drink 1 tablespoon of lemon juice mixed with 1 tablespoon of olive oil every 2 hours for three doses. Eat some bread 1 hour after each dose.

Fractures and sprains
Vitamin C aids collagen production, which means that getting sufficient vitamin C can help the healing of fractured bones of sprained ligaments.

Heal from the inside out
Include the juice of a lemon in your daily diet.

Sunburn
The antioxidants in lemons could discourage sunburn.

Heal from the inside out
Include the zest and juice of a lemon in your daily diet.

Quick fixes
Mix 3 drops of lemon oil into 2 tablespoons of sweet almond or other carrier oil and apply this to your skin.

Alternatively, apply lemon juice directly to the affected area.

Urine infection
If infection is making your urinary tract inflamed and sore, overly acidic urine – for example, from an unhealthy diet – will worsen the pain. The urine's normal pH (acid–alkaline balance) varies from 4.5 to 9, the ideal perhaps being 5.8 to 6.8. The metabolism of lemon juice in the body has a mildly alkalizing effect that can help restore your urine to its normal state.

Heal from the inside out
Consume the juice of half a lemon 2 or 3 times a day.

Athlete's foot
This fungal infection between the toes is often picked up around swimming pools. Anecdotal reports suggest that lemon juice might help.

Quick fix
Soak a cotton pad in lemon juice and apply to the affected area.

Regular treatment
Alternatively, bathe feet in a bowl of water containing 2 tablespoons of lemon juice.

Cold sores

The limonene in a lemon's juice and particularly in its oil has antiviral properties. Lemon oil also helps by excluding air from a sore.

Regular treatment

Apply lemon juice to a cold sore several times a day, using a clean cotton pad each time.

Soothing cold sore treatment

1 drop lemon oil   2 teaspoons sweet almond oil

1   Put the sweet almond oil in a jar and add the lemon oil. Mix together.
2   Use a cotton wool ball to apply the mixture to the cold sore as required.

General infection
Lemon oil has some degree of antibacterial, antiviral and antifungal action, mainly thanks to its limonene and antioxidants. The flavonoid hesperidin may help prevent serious infection.

Heal from the inside out
Include the zest and juice of a lemon in your daily diet.

Coughs and colds

Colds, 'flu and sore throat
There is some scientific backing for the belief that taking at least 1g of vitamin C a day, starting from the first symptoms, reduces the likely length of a cold. However, it actually helps prevent colds only in people who undertake extreme exertion in cold weather (such as skiers). Also, since a lemon contains only around 60–100mg of vitamin C, you would need to consume a lot of lemons!

- The flavonoids in lemons enhance the action of vitamin C. Also, some of them have anti-viral, anti-bacterial and anti-inflammatory properties. Quercetin, for example, has anti-viral properties.
- The water in homemade lemonade (see page 32) helps replace fluid lost in sneezes, catarrh and – if you are feverish – sweat. Water makes catarrh moister and easier to shift, and helps prevent dehydration, which can cause headaches.
- The decongestant vapour of lemon oil can shrink the swollen mucous membrane lining the air passages and

Eustachian tubes. This eases breathing and discourages deafness.

- Another benefit of lemons is that the bowel's bacteria ferment their pectin. This releases butyric acid and other short-chain fatty acids with prebiotic qualities – meaning they nourish 'good' probiotic bowel bacteria such as lactobacilli and bifidobacteria. These, in turn, benefit our immunity.
- A 2005 German study of 479 volunteers found that taking tablets containing lactobacilli and bifidobacteria reduced the severity of colds, shortened their length by two days and increased the number of immune cells.

Heal from the inside out
Drink 3–6 glasses of lemonade (see pages 32–3) each day.
   Add two or three cloves or a small pinch of dried cinnamon to each glass to ease a fever.

Regular treatment
Gargle with 1 teaspoon of lemon juice in a glass of warm water twice a day.

Quick fix
If you have gone deaf, put a few drops of lemon oil on a paper tissue and inhale its vapour.

Soothing cough mixture

Heating linseeds (flax seeds) with lemon will create a warming, soothing drink.

½ lemon   honey, to taste
2 tablespoons cracked linseeds
   (flax seeds)

1   Add 500ml (1 pint) water to a small saucepan.
2   Slice the ½ lemon and add to the pan with the linseeds.
3   Bring to the boil and simmer over a low heat for 20 minutes.
4   Strain the cough mixture into a jug (pitcher) and sweeten with
    honey, to taste.
5   When sufficiently cooled, pour into a cup and drink as
    required.

Essential oils vapour bath

Lemon essential oil is an expectorant, encouraging the airways to expel mucus.

2 drops lemon essential oil   2 drops tea tree oil
2 drops eucalyptus oil

1   Fill a bowl with just-boiled water and place the bowl carefully on a surface that you can sit in front of, such as a kitchen table
2   Add the oils to the water.
3   Sitting down, lean over the bowl, covering your head and the bowl with a towel. Make sure that the towel is large enough so that none of the steam can escape.
4   Inhale the vapour for as long as is comfortable. Repeat as required.

Honey, lemon and ginger tea

This is a classic remedy for coughs and colds.

2.5cm (1 inch) piece of fresh
root ginger

1 tablespoon freshly squeezed
lemon juice
1 tablespoon honey

1   Grate the ginger into a jug (pitcher) or a teapot.
2   Pour 1 cup of boiling water over the ginger and allow to steep
    for 3–5 minutes.
3   Add the lemon juice and honey to a cup or mug.
4   Pour the ginger tea through a strainer into the cup or mug.
5   Stir well to dissolve the honey. Taste, and add more lemon or
    honey as required.

Bronchitis

Chronic bronchitis is an obstructive lung disease that may require ever-more intensive treatment. Anti-inflammatory antioxidants seem to be protective, and quercetin may play a key role. Pectin may help too.

Researchers say that high consumption of fibre and fruit is associated with less coughing. They believe flavonoids are partly responsible.

Heal from the inside out

Include the zest and juice of a lemon in your daily diet.

Women's health

Fibroids

One possible reason for these non-cancerous growths in the womb is an oestrogen/progesterone imbalance. This could activate genes that encourage womb-muscle fibres to proliferate. Another possibility is being very overweight, as fat cells produce oestrogen, and larger women tend to have high levels of blood sugar and growth hormone. A third possibility is pressure on and in the womb from congestion of blood and lymph in the pelvis. The fibre in lemons reduces the numbers of gut bacteria that produce the enzyme beta-glucuronidase, which enables the reabsorption of oestrogen from the bowel into the blood. The B vitamins in lemons encourage the liver to break down surplus oestrogen. And their vitamin C – with help from flavonoids – strengthens tiny blood vessels (capillaries).

Heal from the inside out
Include the zest and juice of a lemon in your daily diet.

Heavy periods
Possible triggers include stress, hormone imbalance, iron deficiency anaemia, inelastic blood vessels due to a poor diet, fibroids, womb infection, and inflammation from a contraceptive device.

Lemon juice is a traditional folk remedy for heavy periods. If it works, it's probably because of some combination of its minerals (such as calcium, iron, magnesium and zinc), vitamins (such as beta-carotene and vitamin C) and flavonoids (such as rutin).

Heal from the inside out
• Include the zest and juice of 2 lemons in your daily diet.

Pre-menstrual syndrome
Pre-menstrual syndrome is probably caused by changes in levels of neurotransmitters, such as serotonin and GABA (gamma-amino butyric acid), resulting from oversensitivity to the changing balance of progesterone and oestrogen during this part of the menstrual cycle. Research suggests that glucaric acid salts help by suppressing the enzyme beta-glucuronidase. This enables a process called glucuronidation in the liver, which makes oestrogen more water-soluble and thus aids its elimination in the urine. Limonene also encourages glucuronidation.

Regular treatment
Include the zest and juice of a lemon in your daily diet during the 2 weeks before you expect a period.

Historically, some women around the Mediterranean aimed to prevent pregnancy by soaking a piece of sea-sponge in a mixture of one part of lemon juice to five parts of water and putting it in their vagina before sex. This would have added to the natural acidity of the vagina. The DNA in sperm is normally protected from being broken down by the vagina's acidity, thanks to substances called amines in seminal fluid, which make semen alkaline. But extra acidity from diluted lemon juice can overwhelm this protection and stop sperm swimming in as short a time as 30 seconds, so they can't get to the egg and fertilize it. However, while this might sound like a useful method of contraception, experts consider it unacceptably unreliable compared with modern methods of contraception.

Oral health

Gingivitis
Antioxidants and other anti-inflammatories in lemons may relieve the pain and swelling of unhealthy gums.

Regular treatment
Massage gums twice a day with lemon juice.

Antiseptic and astringent mouthwash

2 tablespoons cold water
2 tablespoons freshly squeezed
   lemon juice

or

1 cup warm water
1 drop lemon essential oil

1   Mix your chosen ingredients together in a glass or cup.
2   Take a mouthful of the mouthwash and swill around your mouth before spitting out. Repeat several times.

Mouth ulcers

Lemon oil is reputed to ease the pain of aphthous ulcers.

Regular treatment

Apply lemon juice to the affected area several times a day.

Oil treatment for ulcers

3 drops lemon essential oil

3 drops tea tree essential oil

2 drops myrrh essential oil

1 tablespoon sweet almond oil
(or other carrier oil)

1 Mix the ingredients together in a small jar.
2 Apply a few drops of the oil to the mouth ulcer with your finger, every 2 hours.

General health

Headache
Some complementary practitioners believe headaches can result from our body's buffer systems working extra hard to keep the blood's pH (acidity–alkalinity level) within its normal, very slightly alkaline range of 7.35–7.45. Others believe that headaches can result from the blood's pH being at the higher (more alkaline) end of its normal range. They recommend treatment with vinegar. Interestingly, vinegar is a folk remedy familiar from the nursery rhyme in which Jack mends his head with 'vinegar and brown paper'. Lemon juice has similar acidity.

Quick fixes
Sponge your head with lemon juice, or apply a flannel (washcloth) soaked in 570ml/1 pint/2. cups of water containing 2 tablespoons of lemon juice.

Inhale mildly acidic vapour by putting 1 tablespoon of lemon juice into a vaporizer and staying close until it has evaporated.

Regular treatment
Three times a day drink a cup of hot water containing 1 tablespoon of lemon juice.

Infertility
Vitamins B, C and E, folic acid, selenium and zinc in lemons help nourish sperm and eggs and help sperm swim.

Heal from the inside out
Include the zest and juice of a lemon in your daily diet.

Insomnia

Inhaling the vapour of lemon oil is said to have sedative properties.

Regular treatment

Add a few drops of lemon essential oil to your bath water.
Put a few drops of lemon oil on your pillow at bedtime.

Relaxing bedtime massage

2–3 drops lemon essential oil

2–3 drops ylang ylang essential oil (antidepressant, confidence-boosting)

2–3 drops vetivert essential oil (sedative, comforting)

1   Mix the oils together in a small bowl.
2   Before going to bed, lie down, and put a few drops of the mixture on the palm of your hand.
3   Relax, and move your hand around the outer margin of your abdomen in smooth, slow, clockwise circles.

Low immunity

Lemons contain vitamin C, which boosts immunity. In addition, their pectin fibre is degraded by 'good' micro-organisms in the large bowel, liberating short-chain fatty acids, such as butyric acid. These aid immunity by stimulating the production of helper T cells, antibodies, white blood cells and cyto- kines. They also inhibit C-reactive protein, which is a marker of inflammation.

Heal from the inside out

Include the zest and juice of a lemon in your daily diet.

Metabolic syndrome

This is some combination (subject to debate) of high fasting blood glucose levels (pre-diabetes), high blood pressure, an apple-shaped body, low HDL cholesterol and high triglycerides. It encourages diabetes, heart disease and strokes, affects one in five people, and is also known as insulin resistance syndrome or syndrome X. It's more likely with increasing age and can be associated with polycystic ovary syndrome. Most sufferers are sedentary, obese and insulin-resistant. Researchers suspect that inflammation and oxidation play a part. Certainly, affected people are more likely to have a high level of C-reactive protein, indicating inflammation.

Lemon antioxidants and acids may help to prevent prediabetes, high blood pressure, obesity and unhealthy levels of cholesterol and triglycerides.

Heal from the inside out

Include the zest and juice of a lemon in your daily diet.

Fainting

Faints, or dizziness warning of them, can indicate that brain cells lack energy because the blood sugar is low. The acidity and fibre content of lemons slows the absorption of sugar from the gut. This helps prevent blood sugar rising too high then dipping too low. Lemon juice may particularly help those who lack stomach acid (such as one in two over-60s, and certain people who are stressed) and are also 'fast oxidizers' of sugar. Fast oxidizers quickly use up the readily available sugar in their blood, so feel hungry and, perhaps, faint soon after eating. Acidic foods, like stomach acid, promote protein digestion. This enables such people to get energy from protein, so they are less likely to faint.

Heal from the inside out

Include the zest and juice of a lemon in your daily diet.

Fatigue

Lemons supply small amounts of B vitamins, which can ease fatigue. Their fibre slows the absorption of sugar, which steadies blood-sugar levels and helps prevent low-blood-sugar dips, which can trigger fatigue.

Lemon acids could reduce tiredness associated with poor absorption of protein and certain other nutrients due to a lack of stomach acid. Low stomach acid is more likely with ageing, stress, prolonged use of acid-suppressant medication and a diet high in meat, grain, sugar and carbonated drinks (which produce acid in the body) but low in vegetables and fruits. A lemon's acidity could aid digestion by lowering the pH of the stomach. What's more, some alternative practitioners say, though without proof, that a deficiency in sodium from fruits and vegetables encourages the body to divert sodium from stomach-acid-producing cells so it's available to 'partner' acids in the urine. They say this could prevent the proper production of stomach acid. The sodium from lemons, though present in very small amounts, could help.

Heal from the inside out
Include the zest and juice of a lemon in your daily diet.

Muscle stiffness
Pain and stiffness experienced after exercise might respond to anti-inflammatories such as nobiletin in lemon oil.

Quick fix
Put 1 teaspoon of lemon oil in your bathwater and relax for half an hour.

Muscle relaxer

3 drops lemon oil

2–3 drops ginger oil (an
analgesic and local circulation
booster)

3 tablespoons sweet almond oil
(or other carrier oil)

1   Mix the oils together in a small bowl.
2   Massage the affected muscles in a circular motion with the oil
mixture.

Neuralgia

The cooling and anti-inflammatory properties of lemon juice may ease pain from an irritated nerve.

Regular treatment

Apply warmed lemon juice over the painful area and repeat each hour for half a day.

Quick fixes

Add 3 drops of lemon oil to 2 tablespoons of sweet almond or other carrier oil, and smooth over the affected area.

Add a few drops of lemon oil to the water in an aromatherapy diffuser, or put them in a bowl of just-boiled water and lean over it with a towel over your head, to inhale the vapour.

Piles

Piles are spongy pads in the walls of the anus (back passage) that have become bulky and loose. They readily become inflamed, and inflammation can cause discomfort, itching and bleeding. Causes include constipation and fragile veins. Lemons can help, as their vitamin C and rutin and certain other flavonoids strengthen veins; their fibre helps prevent constipation; and their anti-inflammatory antioxidants reduce inflammation.

Heal from the inside out

Include the zest and juice of a lemon in your daily diet.

Restlessness

Lemons might help, as they contain the flavonoid hesperidin. Hesperidin can act as a sedative, possibly via action on the body's opioid or adenosine receptors.

Heal from the inside out
Include the zest and juice of a lemon in your daily diet.

Varicose veins
Lemons can act as a venous tonic as they have strengthening, astringent and anti-inflammatory effects on vein walls.

Heal from the inside out
Include the zest and juice of a lemon in your daily diet.

Anti-inflammatory massage oil

2 drops lemon essential oil

2 drops lavender essential oil

3 drops cypress essential oil

2 tablespoons sweet almond oil (or other carrier oil)

1   Mix the oils together in a small bowl.

2   Massage your legs with oil, paying particular attention to areas affected by varicose veins.

Long-term/serious conditions

Chronic illness

This can indicate a need for antioxidants such as vitamin C. Lemons are an excellent source and their flavonoids enhance the action of their vitamin C.

Lemon acids could help if you also have insufficient stomach acid and therefore poor absorption of certain nutrients. Low stomach acid affects one in two over-60s and can result from ageing, stress, the prolonged use of acid-suppressant medication, and an unhealthy diet high in meat, grain, sugar and carbonated drinks (which produce acid in the body) and low in vegetables and fruits. A lemon's acidity could aid digestion by lowering the pH of the stomach. Some alternative practitioners say, though without proof, that a deficiency of sodium from fruits and vegetables encourages the body to divert sodium from stomach-acid producing cells, so it's available to 'partner' acids in the urine and let them escape from the body. They say this could reduce the production of stomach acid.

Heal from the inside out

Include the zest and juice of a lemon in your daily diet.

Diabetes

The raised blood sugar of pre-diabetes encourages diabetes, whilst untreated or poorly treated diabetes encourages heart, eye and kidney disease. Lemons might help in several ways.

Acid-containing foods seem very useful. Studies suggest that vinegar helps prevent high blood sugar. Experts believe that vinegar reduces a meal's 'glycaemic index' (ability to raise blood sugar) and that it delays stomach emptying, inactivates intestinal enzymes that convert complex sugars to glucose, and reduces the production and release of sugar from non-carbohydrate sources in the liver. Lemon juice, like other acidic foods, behaves in a similar way. Indeed, certain acidic foods have as powerful an effect on a meal's glycaemic index as the diabetes drug metformin.

Frequent consumption of acidic foods is traditional in many countries and may help explain national variations in the rate of diabetes.

A lemon's fibre may help, too. 'Good' bowel bacteria break down pectin, liberating short-chain fatty acids, such as butyric acid, which reduce the release of sugar from the liver's stores. Short-chain fatty acids also inhibit C-reactive protein – a blood marker of inflammation and a predictor of diabetes.

Heal from the inside out
Include the zest and juice of a lemon in your daily diet.

Cancer
Cancer results from mutation of a cell's DNA (genetic material). This produces malignant cells – meaning ones that continue multiplying instead of dying (from apoptosis – 'cell suicide') at their allotted time. A lack of antioxidants encourages certain cancers. These normally mop up free radicals (unstable particles), which are continually produced in the body and can encourage cancer by damaging a cell's DNA. Lemons – and especially their peel – contain almost every known type of cancer-preventing and cancer-fighting phytochemical, including

carotenoids, flavonoids, limonene, pectin, glucaric acid
salts, and terpenes.

Research suggests that:
- The flavonoid tangeretin helps prevent cancer growth by
  disturbing signalling between tumour cells.
- The flavonoid nobiletin can kill cancer cells, help prevent
  breast and colon cancers and certain leukaemias by
  inducing apoptosis of malignant cells, and make cancer
  cells less resistant to chemotherapy.
- The flavonoids naringenin and quercetin inhibit liver
  enzymes that convert the tobacco-related substance
  NNK into a potent inducer of lung cancer.
- Coumarins discourage cancer growth.
- Limonene helps prevent breast and colon cancers.
- Limonoids help fight cancers of the mouth, skin, lung,
  breast, stomach and colon.
- Glucaric acid salts discourage bowel cancer by promoting
  the production in the gut of butyric acid, which
  encourages apoptosis of malignant cells.
- Pectin's prebiotic properties help colon cells produce
  mucus, which helps stop carcinogens sticking to the
  gut lining.
- Pectin reduces the progression of advanced prostate
  cancer and makes mouth and throat cancers less likely to
  recur.

Researchers have found that regular consumption of black
tea containing lemon zest is associated with a reduction in
skin-cancer risk of more than 70 per cent, black tea alone
with a 40 per-cent reduction.

A US study has linked a citrus-rich diet with a reduction in stomach cancer in men.

Some alternative practitioners believe that our diet can influence cancer by affecting the metabolic processes that keep our body's pH (acid–alkaline) balance within its normal tightly controlled range. However, although cancerous tissue certainly may be unusually acidic, there is currently little evidence to support this view.

Heart disease

The most common sort of heart disease – coronary artery disease – involves atherosclerosis, in which artery-lining (endothelial) cells leak, allowing penetration by lipids such as LDL-cholesterol and triglycerides. The lipids are then oxidized by free radicals, attracting white blood cells, which cause inflammation. Smooth-muscle cells produce collagen to cover leaks in the lining, and calcium infiltrates affected areas. All this stiffens blood vessels and prevents them from expanding and contracting as they should. It also forms plaques, which can rupture, causing clots that can trigger a heart attack. (Atherosclerosis can affect arteries elsewhere too; in the brain, for example, they encourage a stroke.)

Lemons can help many of the risk factors for coronary artery disease. They can reduce obesity, high blood pressure, diabetes, and high cholesterol, homocysteine (via their folate) and C-reactive protein (via their anti-inflammatories). Lemons can also reduce the oxidation associated with smoking and stress (via their antioxidants).

Studies suggest that flavonoids (as in lemon peel) discourage heart disease.

'Good' micro-organisms in the bowel degrade pectin from lemons, freeing short-chain fatty acids such as butyric acid. These reduce LDL cholesterol, increase HDL cholesterol (the potentially protective sort) and inhibit C-reactive protein.

Heal from the inside out
Include the zest and juice of a lemon in your daily diet.

High blood pressure
Lemons can affect several of the risk factors, which include obesity, age, insulin resistance (pre-diabetes), salt sensitivity, and overactivity of the kidney hormone renin. First, they encourage weight loss. Second, their potassium helps regulate body fluids, their magnesium relaxes arteries, their fibre encourages weight loss, their flavonoids promote arterial health and their acids discourage pre-diabetes. In many people, fatty, chalky atheroma builds up in artery walls. Free radicals (encouraged by a poor diet, infection, smoking, stress) oxidize LDL cholesterol in atheroma, and trigger immune cells to inflame arteries. Atheroma and inflammation together stiffen the arteries, encouraging high blood pressure. Russian folklore recommends lemon and orange juice to help prevent this.

Heal from the inside out
Include the zest and juice of a lemon in your daily diet.

High cholesterol
An unhealthy diet and insufficient exercise and sunlight encourage too much LDL (low density lipoprotein) cholesterol in the blood, plus too little HDL (high density lipoprotein) cholesterol, and high levels of total cholesterol and triglycerides (types of fats now properly

called triacylglycerols). The liver makes 80 per cent of the body's cholesterol from triglycerides and a substance called apolipoprotein B. Various constituents of lemons can influence this production. Oxidation of LDL cholesterol by free radicals (enhanced by stress, sunlight, exercise and smoking) encourages high blood pressure, heart attacks and strokes. The vitamin C, phenolic compounds (including flavonoids), pectin, limonin and acids in lemons encourage healthy cholesterol levels.

Pectin thickens the bowel contents, which reduces the absorption of cholesterol from food and bile and helps eliminate it. Also, 'good' gut bacteria degrade pectin, liberating short- chain fatty acids such as butyric acid, which inhibit cholesterol absorption, suppress its production in the liver, and boost HDL cholesterol.

Studies show that pectin plus vitamin C lowers cholesterol more than pectin alone, and pectin plus phenolic compounds lower cholesterol and triglycerides more than either alone.

Lemons are richer than apples in pectin. Eating one large apple each day lowers cholesterol by up to 11 per cent; two lower it by up to 16 per cent; and four have the cholesterol-lowering power of a statin drug!

Researchers at Florida University found that giving pectin to pigs reduced cholesterol by 30 per cent and reduced expected arterial calcification.

The US Agricultural Research Service found that liver cells produce less of the protein apo B (needed to make LDL cholesterol) when exposed to limonin.

Alternative practitioners claim that a healthy diet containing plenty of 'alkaline-forming' foods, such as lemons, helps dissolve and eliminate cholesterol.

Research suggests that a lemon's glucaric acid salts reduce LDL cholesterol by up to 35 per cent.

Heal from the inside out
Include the zest and juice of 1 or 2 lemons in your daily diet

Strokes
A stroke ('brain attack') usually results from a blood clot interrupting the blood flow in one of the brain's arteries (when it's called a thrombotic stroke). Less often it's caused by bleeding in the brain from an unhealthy artery (a haemorrhagic stroke).

The main culprits behind a thrombotic stroke are the narrowing, roughening and inflammation of an artery in the brain by atheroma (see Heart disease, page 107). Clots readily form in affected arteries, especially if there are also other risk factors, such as smoking, stress, an unhealthy diet, obesity, high blood pressure, diabetes and chronic infection. Lemons can help many of the risk factors for strokes. They can help reduce obesity, high blood pressure, diabetes and high cholesterol, homocysteine (via their folate) and C-reactive protein (via their anti-inflammatories). Lemons can also reduce the oxidation associated with smoking and stress (via their anti-oxidants). The vitamin C and flavonoids in lemons may discourage several possible causes of strokes.

Research suggests that flavonoids in lemon peel help prevent oxidation of LDL cholesterol. Flavonoids are also thought to reduce cholesterol production in the liver. Studies suggest that flavonoids improve the behaviour of artery-lining cells and help prevent blood clots. 'Good' micro-organisms in the bowel degrade pectin from lemons, freeing short-chain fatty acids such as butyric acid. These reduce LDL cholesterol, increase HDL cholesterol (the potentially protective sort) and inhibit C-reactive protein.

Heal from the inside out
Include the zest and juice of a lemon in your daily diet.

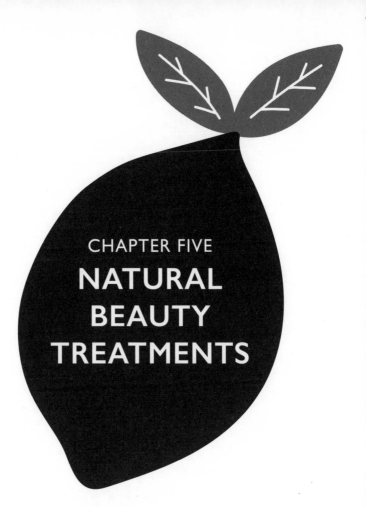

CHAPTER FIVE

NATURAL BEAUTY TREATMENTS

5

NATURAL BEAUTY TREATMENTS

Every part of a lemon contains beautifying ingredients. Lemon juice can cleanse, soften and moisturize your skin, condition and lighten your hair and deodorize your body. Lemon oil is moisturizing and toning. It also has a light, fresh, appealing fragrance that can lift the spirits, and when diluted with a carrier oil it is lovely for a massage.

Another reason why lemon juice is such a good beauty aid is that its organic acids can help maintain or restore the skin's natural acidity.

Normal skin has a slightly acidic surface layer called the acid mantle or hydro-lipid film. This contains:

- the fats (lipids) of skin oil (sebum)
- the lactic acid and amino acids of sweat
- the amino acids and pyrrolidine carboxylic acid of dead skin cells

The skin's normal pH (acid/alkaline balance) over most of the body in women is 4.5–5.75 (below 7 on this scale is acidic, above is alkaline). Men's skin is slightly more acidic. This slight acidity helps repair damaged skin and activates enzymes that enable the production of lipids in sebum. This helps explain why water finds it hard to escape from the skin (other than in perspiration) and harmful substances and micro-organisms find it hard to enter. It also encourages healthy populations of bacteria and fungi on the skin and helps prevent infection. Reduced acidity – caused, for example, by most soaps, and by eczema or other dermatitis – encourages drying, cracking and itching.

Most soaps, even mild, glycerine or baby ones and beauty bars, have an alkaline pH of 7–9, which temporarily destroys the skin's normal acidity. In healthy skin, the acidity generally recovers between 30 minutes and two hours (or more), though twice-daily soaping compromises this degree of restoration. Certain soaps are particularly alkaline (pH 9.5–11). The pH of Dove soap is relatively low at 6.5–7.5, but only a very few bar soaps (for example, Cetaphil and Aquaderm) have a pH similar to that of normal skin. However, the pH of many liquid soaps, non-soap cleansers and bath and shower gels resembles that of normal skin more closely; and the pH of a few (for example, Johnsons pH 5.5 Hand Wash) is similar to that of normal skin.

Using a cleanser containing lemon juice avoids any reduction in acidity. Or, if you want to use alkaline soap, you can rinse your skin afterwards with a 'splash' of diluted lemon juice.

Lemon acids are moisturizing. This is partly because they help maintain or restore the skin's acidity, which helps prevent water loss, and partly because a lemon's citric acid is an alpha-hydroxy acid, meaning it has an intrinsic moisturizing action. It also loosens dead skin cells and encourages them to flake off. So it can soften and smooth rough or hard skin and help cracked skin to heal. The softening produced by citric acid helps explain why applying lemon juice makes blackheads easier to remove with gentle fingertip pressure or a blackhead extractor. What's more, the astringent properties of lemon juice tend to contract large pores, so there's less space for blackheads in them. Also, the vitamin C and other antioxidants in lemon juice help prevent lipids in sebum from being oxidized and therefore blackened by air to create a blackhead.

CITRIC ACID

This is one of the alpha hydroxy acids (AHAs) beloved of beauty-product manufacturers. Skin products containing AHAs have moisturizing and exfoliating properties, as they help the skin retain water and encourage the separation of dead skin cells. This explains why applying lemon juice can moisturize dry skin and restore softness and smoothness to hard, cracked or flaking skin.

Rutin and certain other flavonoids in lemons can strengthen the walls of the capillaries, our tiniest blood vessels. So including the zest and juice of a lemon in your daily diet could help prevent the tiny broken veins that sometimes occur on the face and elsewhere.

The moisturizing and softening properties of its acids make lemon juice an excellent aid for a manicure or pedicure.

Diluted lemon juice also restores acidity to just-washed hair. Most shampoos are alkaline, so they temporarily destroy the scalp's normal acidity, leaving it prone to dryness, irritation and even infection. Their residues also dull the hair. A lemon rinse not only makes hair shine but can also enhance natural highlights.

Caution: Avoid putting neat lemon oil on your skin within 12 hours before sunlight exposure. Or use no more than one drop per 2 teaspoons of sweet almond or other carrier oil, so it's unlikely to trigger a photosensitive reaction.

Daily routine

It's easy to add homemade lemon products to your everyday skincare routine. Use these remedies to cleanse, tone and moisturize yourself to better, more healthy and more naturally radiant skin.

Herby lemon steam cleanser

900ml/30fl oz/3. cups water
full-thickness peel of half a
  lemon
1 teaspoon dried mint (or 2
  teaspoons chopped fresh
  mint)

1 teaspoon dried parsley
  (2 teaspoons chopped fresh
  parsley)
contents of a capsule of evening
  primrose oil (optional, for
  dry skin)

1   Pour the water into a saucepan and bring to the boil.
2   Transfer the just-boiled water to a bowl and add the lemon
    peel, mint, parsley and evening primrose oil, if using. Mix
    together well.
3   Sit for at least 5 minutes with your face over the bowl and a
    towel over both your head and the bowl.
4   Rinse your face with lukewarm water.

Chilled lemon toner

juice of I lemon   cold water

1   Put the lemon juice into a jar or bottle.
2   Add twice its volume of water to the jar or bottle.
3   Place in the refrigerator for 1–2 hours, until chilled.
4   After cleansing your face, apply some of this lemon toner with
    a cotton pad and leave to dry naturally.

Quick and easy moisturizer
Smooth lemon juice over your skin, wait for half an hour, then rinse.

Natural deodorant
Because it has antibacterial properties, lemon juice can act as a deodorant.

Rub the cut surface of a lemon over each armpit or simply add the juice of a lemon to your bath water.

Home SPA treatments
We all need to indulge in a little self-care sometimes. Taking care of our bodies with indulgent treatments can work wonders on our mental health, too. Try these ideas to help you relax, unwind and reap all the natural benefits of lemons.

Exfoliating bath salts

225g/8oz/¾ cup of sea salt   ½ teaspoon lemon essential oil

1   Make lemon-scented salt by putting the sea salt into a bowl.
     Stir in the lemon essential oil and transfer the mixture to a
     screw-top jar.
2   Get rid of dead skin cells by rubbing damp skin with the
     lemon-scented salt while enjoying a warm bath.

Anti-ageing face mask

I egg

I tablespoon lemon juice

I drop of vitamin E oil from a
capsule

1   Separate the egg yolk from the white, putting each into a
    different small bowl.
2   Add 1 teaspoon of egg yolk to the white, and stir together to
    combine.
3   Add the lemon juice and vitamin E oil and mix again.
4   To smooth fine lines and wrinkles, apply the mask to your face,
    then lie down for half an hour.
5   Wash and dry your skin and apply moisturizer.

Rejuvenating banana treatment

1 ripe banana   1 teaspoon honey
1 teaspoon lemon juice

1   Peel the banana and place in a small bowl. Mash with a fork.
2   Add the lemon juice and honey and mash again, making
    sure everything is nicely combined. Ensure that there are no
    large lumps.
3   Apply to your skin in an even layer and relax for 10 minutes.
4   Wash off with warm water and pat your face dry with a towel.

Brightening turmeric mask

1 teaspoon plain yogurt

1 tablespoon lemon juice

1 tablespoon honey

½ teaspoon ground turmeric

1 Place all the ingredients together in a small bowl, mixing well to combine.

2 Smooth the mask over your skin in an even layer and relax for 15–20 minutes.

3 Remove the mask with warm water and pat your face dry with a towel.

Manicure or pedicure

½ lemon   warm water

1   Squeeze the juice from the ½ lemon into a bowl, reserving
    the peel.
2   Pour warm water over the lemon juice, and soften cuticles and
    whiten stained hands and nails by soaking them for 10 minutes
3   Gently push back your cuticles.
4   Rub a strip of the reserved lemon peel on your nails to make
    them shine.

FINGERTIP SPLITS

Splits in the skin at the ends of your fingertips are surprisingly painful. Lemon essential oil can soothe the pain, soften the hard edges of cut skin and speed healing. Dig the fingertip into the under-surface of some lemon rind. This opens the lemon-oil glands and releases oil on to the split skin. Repeat two or three times a day until better.

Problem areas

- To soften hard skin on the elbows, sit with each one in a squeezed-out half-lemon shell for 30 minutes.
- To treat existing blackheads and prevent further outbreaks, smooth lemon juice over the affected skin and let it dry. Repeat each day as necessary.
- To aid with broken veins, consume the zest and juice of a lemon each day to provide your veins with strengthening rutin and other flavonoids.

Massage

Lemon oil blends well with many other essential oils, including lavender, rose, neroli, sandalwood, geranium and ylang ylang, to create a soothing massage oil. Experiment with different combinations until you find a few that work for you.

Mix a few drops of each essential oil with a couple of tablespoons of sweet almond oil, or another carrier oil of your choice.

A lemon's wonderful complex fragrance results from the combination of the fragrances of its many scented components. These are mainly terpenes (many of whose names end in 'ene') and their derivatives – including various alcohols (whose names end in 'ol') and aldehydes (whose names end in 'al'). There are also various coumarins and unsaturated fatty acids. The compounds that contribute most to a lemon's odour are citral, limonene, pinene and terpinene. One of the main reasons for the difference in scent of various lemon oils is their ratio of citral to citronellal.

A lemon's fragrance components include:

- bergamotene (black pepper)
- bisabolene (sweet, spicy, balsamic)
- cadinene (woody)
- camphene (pungent)
- caryophyllene (musky, oriental, sandalwood)
- citral (lemon)
- citronellal ('green', citrus)
- decanal (orange)
- dipentene (pine, lime, herbal, lemon)
- farnesenes (apple)
- geranial (strong lemon)
- geraniol (rose)
- heptanal (fresh, 'green', citrus)
- hexanol (herbaceous, woody)
- limonene (orange)
- linalool (sweet, woody, lavender)
- methyl anthranilate (grape)
- myrcene (woody)

- neral (sweet lemon)
- nerol (sweet rose)
- nonanol (fresh, spicy, herbaceous)
- nootkatone ('green', grapefruit)
- octanal (citrus)
- paracymene (fresh, citrus, woody, spicy)
- phellandrene (peppery, minty, citrus)
- pinene (pine, resinous)
- sabinene (marjoram)
- scopoletin (oaky, nutty)
- terpinene ('green', citrus)
- terpineol (lilac)
- umbelliferone (woody, medicinal)

Other plants with a lemon scent or flavour include lemon balm, lemon geranium, lemon grass, lemon myrtle, lemon verbena and lemon-scented varieties of basil, mint and thyme.

Hair care

Lemon can be used in treatments to suit every hair type. It is a natural bleach, so if you are happy with the colour of your hair, be careful not to use too much when you are going to be spending time in the sun.

Greasy hair

After shampooing greasy hair, rinse with water plus a squeeze of lemon juice. Its acidity counteracts dullness by reducing the alkalinity of traces of shampoo. It also dissolves soap residues that were in the shampoo, which in turn releases fatty acids. All this gives hair an attractive shine and texture.

Dry hair

Similarly, after shampooing dry hair, rinse with water plus a squeeze of lemon juice. Like many commercial dry-haircare products, this contains an organic acid (citric acid), which chelates ('binds') unwanted traces of heavy metals and shampoo that can further dry the hair.

Coloured hair

After bleaching or colouring your hair, rinse with water containing a squeeze of lemon juice. Lemon acids precipitate proteins, which helps counteract hair damage caused by the bleach or colouring agent.

DIY highlights

185ml/6fl oz/¾ cup of water   4 tablespoons of lemon juice

1   Mix the lemon juice and water together in a jug (pitcher).
2   Rinse clean wet hair with the mixture. Sit in the sun until your
    hair dries, for a sun-kissed effect.

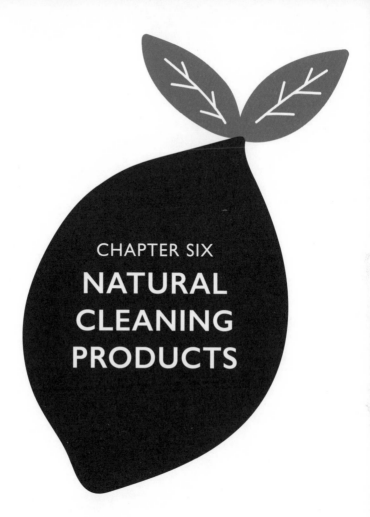

CHAPTER SIX

NATURAL CLEANING PRODUCTS

NATURAL CLEANING PRODUCTS

Lemons are useful for many household chores and can help keep your home clean and sparkling. Making your own cleaning products may seem like a lot of work, but many of the suggestions in this chapter are extremely quick and easy, and use everyday ingredients that you will most likely find you already have in your storecupboard.

Making your own products is fun, and quite addictive. It will allow you to take control over your own environment, as well as saving you money. We all have busy lives, and it may seem easier to pick up a different brightly-coloured bottle for each of your household chores, but consider the benefits of leaving them behind in the store.

Greater control

Store-bought products often contain a cocktail of harsh chemicals which can be absorbed into the skin and breathed in. By making your own products you can be sure that only safe, natural ingredients are being used. You can also control the strength of the product by diluting as required, meaning that you can use the same product at different strengths for different tasks around the home.

More cost effective

Many of the ingredients used in natural cleaning products are easily available and inexpensive. The most commonly used ingredients storecupboard staples like lemons, vinegar and baking soda (bicarbonate of soda).

Environmentally friendly

The use of natural products is often referred to as 'green cleaning'. Making your own products cuts out the levels of pollution that are made during the production of commercial cleaning products, as well as reducing plastic consumption. Not all of the packaging for store-bought cleaning products is recyclable. Some commercial cleaning products may contain ingredients that are tested on animals.

Safer for pets and children

If you know that there are no 'nasties' in your cleaning products, you do not need to worry so much about other family members – especially pets and children – accidentally coming into contact with them. This also applies to any family members who might suffer from allergies – homemade natural products are unlikely to cause asthma attacks or irritation to the skin and eyes.

Create a nicer atmosphere

Homemade products that contain essential oils may have additional beneficial effects on your mood. Think of it as combining a deep cleaning session with an aromatherapy treatment for the whole family!

Using lemons in natural cleaning products

Lemon juice is one of the most effective natural cleaning agents. It contains high levels of citric acid, and has a low pH level as well as antibacterial properties. Note that it is fine to use bottled lemon juice instead of fresh lemon juice for household tasks. This is available from most grocery stores and is very useful to have to hand.

- Before cleaning any area with your homemade lemon products, test a small area first.
- Lemon juice may damage natural stone and brass-plated objects.

Air-freshening

Lemon has a pleasing smell and its scent is used in many commercial cleaning products. It can be used on its own, or in combination with other natural ingredients, to get rid of a variety of unpleasant or unwanted smells around the home.

Mood lifter

Half-fill the bowl of a ceramic diffuser with water, add a few drops of lemon essential oil (Citrus limonum) and light the nightlight (tea light). The vapour of the oil is said to help lift the spirits, clear the mind and improve concentration.

Room spritzer

Add a few drops of lemon essential oil to a spray bottle half-filled with water, shake well and spray to make the air in a room smell fragrant.

Wardrobe freshener

Leave thinly pared strips of lemon peel to dry out well over several days, then put them in your wardrobe or chest of drawers to scent your clothes.

Pot pourri

Add strips of dried lemon peel to a bowl of fragrant dried flowers or leaves for a pot pourri to scent a room. Sprinkle the contents of the bowl every couple of weeks with a few drops of lemon essential oil to refresh the aroma.

Pomander

Make a wonderfully scented pomander by studding a lemon with cloves, then tying some ribbon around it so you can hang it up.

Kitchen deodorant
Deodorize the drain of your kitchen sink by putting the juice of a lemon into a glass of water and pouring the lemon water down the plughole.

After cooking
Remove the odour of fish, onion or garlic from your hands by rubbing them with fresh lemon juice.

Vacuum clean
Freshen your vacuum-cleaner bag by sprinkling a few drops of lemon essential oil on to a paper tissue and putting this into the bag.

Cool down
Keep your fridge smelling sweet by putting half a lemon on a saucer.

Fresh air
Make your air humidifier smell good by adding a few drops of lemon juice to its water container.

Dispose of odour
Make a waste-disposal (garbage disposal) unit smell fresh by putting the peel of a lemon through it and rinsing with water.

Carpet freshener

As well as removing any stale or unpleasant smells from carpets and rugs around the house, the essential oils in this vacuum powder will add a calming and relaxing scent wherever it is used.

10 drops lemon essential oil
10 drops lavender essential oil

125g/4½oz/1 cup baking soda (bicarbonate of soda)

1   Place the baking soda (bicarbonate of soda) in a container with a lid. Add the essential oils and mix well.
2   Cover and leave overnight, so that the baking soda (bicarbonate of soda) fully absorbs the oil.
3   To use, sprinkle the mixture generously over the carpet or rug, then vacuum up the powder.

Cleaning

The acidic properties in lemon juice means it is perfect for cutting through dirt, grease and grime in many different areas of the home.

Surface cleaner

Use lemon essential oil to clean kitchen and bathroom surfaces, as its limonene is a solvent that removes greasy marks as well as alcohol does.

Grease be gone

Remove greasy marks from surfaces by applying lemon juice, then rinsing off with a damp cloth.

Limescale treatment

To remove limescale from around a plughole or tap, rub with the cut end of half a lemon, then rinse.

Window cleaner

To clean windows, rub the cut surfaces of a lemon quarter over the glass, wipe off with a damp cloth, then dry with a dry cloth.

Grout whitener

Use an old toothbrush dipped in lemon juice to clean grout between kitchen or bathroom tiles.

Barbecue cleaner

Remove caked-on food residue from barbecue grills and grates with a mixture of lemon juice and salt.

Washing up booster

Add a few drops of lemon juice to washing-up liquid to increase its degreasing properties.

Descaler for kettles and coffee pots

Remove scaly build up inside kettles and coffee pots by adding a few lemon slices to the water and boiling. Once boiled, allow the lemon water to cool down and sit for 1–2 hours, before rinsing out with clean water.

Quick floor cleaner

Add 4 tablespoons of white vinegar and 10 drops of lemon essential oil to a bucket of water and mop the floor with this scented solution.

Scented floor cleaner

Use this fresh smelling floor cleaner on wooden, laminate or ceramic-tiled floors (but not natural stone).

240ml/8fl oz/1 cup of white vinegar

240ml/8fl oz/1 cup of water

5 drops of lemon essential oil

2 drops of tea tree essential oil

5 drops of lavender essential oil

1 Add the vinegar and water to an empty spray bottle and mix together.
2 Add the essential oils and mix once more.
3 To use, spray the mixture on to the floor and wipe clean with a microfibre cloth or a mop.

Microwave deodorizer

This solution can be used to clean and remove unwanted smells from a microwave oven.

30g/1oz/¼ cup of baking soda (bicarbonate of soda)

1 teaspoon white vinegar
6 drops lemon essential oil

1   In a small bowl, mix together all the ingredients to a paste.
2   To use, apply the paste generously to the inside of the microwave with a clean sponge.
3   Rinse with water and leave the microwave door open for 15 minutes to allow for drying, before using.

Polishing

Add sparkle and shine, and a fresh lemony scent, to grubby surfaces around the house.

Surface polish

Use lemon essential oil to polish surfaces, as its limonene acts as a solvent, dissolving old wax, fingerprints and grime.

Shine and buff

Polish dulled surfaces of aluminium or chrome objects by rubbing with the cut surface of half a lemon, then buffing with a cloth.

Copper cleaner

Brighten copper cookware or ornaments. The lemon acids dissolve the tarnish, and the salt, baking soda (bicarbonate of soda) or baking powder act as a mild abrasive to clear it away.

½ lemon

1 tablespoon salt, baking soda (bicarbonate of soda) or baking powder

1   Put the tablespoon of salt, baking soda (bicarbonate of soda) or baking powder onto a saucer or plate.
2   Dip the half a lemon into the powder.
3   To use, rub the lemon over the surface. Rinse with water and dry with a cloth or a paper towel.

Furniture polish

Use this on wooden furniture. The polish accentuates the beauty of the wood; it also nourishes it and prevents it from drying out.

4 tablespoons olive oil

2 tablespoons strained fresh lemon juice

1   Combine the ingredients in a glass jar.
2   To use, apply to furniture by rubbing it in with a clean, dry cloth.

Disinfecting

Lemon juice has antibacterial properties so excels as a natural disinfectant which is safe to use around the whole family,

Water cleanser

Add a squeeze of lemon juice to disinfect drinking water that you think might be contaminated with bacteria.

Antibacterial surface cleaner

Use lemon essential oil to clean kitchen, bathroom and other surfaces that are likely to be contaminated with bacteria. Several of its constituents, including limonene, have antibacterial properties.

Chopping board rinse

Disinfect kitchen chopping boards with lemon juice, as it contains citric and other acids, and bacteria dislike an acidic environment.

Stain removal

The acidity in lemon juice makes it a natural bleach, and as such it can be used to remove unsightly stains from clothing, upholstery, surfaces and even the skin.

Remove cooking stains

If your hands are stained (for example, after peeling onions), rub them with lemon juice to remove the stains.

Clean sweat patches

To remove sweat stains from clothes, scrub gently with half and half lemon juice and water.

Boost washing-machine hot wash

For stains on fabrics that can be washed in hot water, pour 240ml/8fl oz/1 cup of lemon juice into the washing machine during the wash cycle.

Bleach out rust or mildew

To remove rust spots or mildew stains on washable clothing, sprinkle the area generously with salt, then squeeze fresh lemon juice over it. Leave the item for several hours, ideally in direct sunlight. Keep the stain moist by applying more lemon juice as necessary. Brush off the salt and then launder as usual. (Be warned – putting household bleach on rust spots will set the stain.)

Fade fruit stains

Sprinkle lemon juice over berry stains on clothing or other fabric, to help them fade.

Refresh plastic containers

Mix 1 tablespoon of baking soda (bicarbonate of soda) with a few drops of fresh lemon juice to form a paste, then rub this over stains on plastic food-storage containers.

Shower cleaner

Remove the stains left by hard water on glass shower doors or partitions by rubbing with half a lemon.

Clean worktops

Leave fresh lemon juice for 45 minutes on stains on Formica worktops. Then sprinkle with baking soda (bicarbonate of soda), scrub gently and rinse.

Refresh whites

To remove stains from white laundry.

1 tablespoon lemon juice   1 tablespoon cream of tartar

1   Mix the ingredients together in a small bowl.
2   To use, apply the mixture to the stain. Leave for a few minutes, then rinse off with water.

For persistent or extensive staining on a fabric that is washable in very hot water, boil the item in a pan containing 5 tablespoons of cream of tartar to every 1.1 litre/2 pints/4½ cups of water, then rinse.

Dealing with insects

As well as cleaning the home, lemon can be used to get rid of insect infestations, and prevent them from coming back.

Natural insecticide

If kitchen or other cupboards are infested with insects, wipe them with lemon essential oil on a cloth. Its limonene is toxic to insects but not to humans.

Ant repellent

Use a rotten lemon to repel ants.

Moth deterrent

Put strips of dried lemon peel into a little muslin bag and place in cupboards and drawers to repel clothes moths.

Insect prevention

Sprinkle lemon juice around door thresholds and on windowsills, as its scent will deter the entry of insects.

RESOURCES

Here are some of the organizations concerned with lemons and lemon products around the world.

United Kingdom
Global Orange Groves UK
www.globalorangegroves.co.uk
This nursery offers a variety of
citrus trees, including several
types of lemon, that are
suitable for growing in the UK.

United States
USDA (United States
Department of Agriculture)
www.usda.gov
Provides information on lemons
and lemon juice.

Florida Citrus Information
www.UltimateCitrus.com
Provides links to various sites
associated with the citrus
industry in Florida.

Australia
Citrus Australia (formerly
Australian Citrus Growers)
www.citrusaustralia.com.au
Represents citrus growers in
Australia.

New Zealand
New Zealand Citrus Growers
Incorporated
www.citrus.co.nz
Promotes the interests of citrus
growers and the sustainable
growth and profitability of
the citrus industry in New
Zealand.

Argentina
Tucuman Citrus Association
www.atcitrus.com
Represents the citrus industry
in Argentina, including
producers, packers,
manufacturers and exporters.

South Africa
Citrus Growers Association of
Southern Africa
www.cga.co.za
Represents producers of export
citrus fruit throughout
Southern Africa, including
Zimbabwe and Swaziland.

INDEX

acetic acid 69–70

acid reflux 28

acid–alkaline balance 24
   and ageing 69–70, 71
   and anxiety 67
   and headaches 94
   and kidney stones 62
   and osteoporosis 73–4
   and the skin 115–18
   and urine infections 80

acidity of lemons x, 6, 15, 23–25
   and age-related problems 73–4
   and chronic illness 104, 109
   and cooking 36
   and digestive problems 57–59,
      61–3, 64
   and first aid 78–9
   and general health 97, 98
   and haircare 131
   and the skin 115, 116
   and tooth enamel 50
   and women's health 90
   see also specific acids

acne 50–1

age spots 51

age-related conditions 21, 69–75,
   71

age-related macular degeneration
   (AMD) 71

ageing 19, 69–70

air-freshening 140–2, 146

alcohols 26, 129

aldehydes 26, 28, 129

alkalinizing properties 23, 62, 73,
   80, 109

allergens 21

allergies 50, 61–2, 76–7

alpha hydroxy acids (AHAs) 24,
   116, 117

Alzheimer's disease 69, 70, 74–5

AMD *see* age-related macular
   degeneration

amines 36, 90

amino acids 64, 74

amyloid protein 74

anaemia 57–8
   iron-deficiency 57
   vitamin B12-deficiency 57

ankle swelling 65

anti-cancer agents 28

anti-dandruff treatments 56

anti-inflammatories 20, 26, 83
   and age-related diseases 73–5
   anti-inflammatory massage oil
      103
   and general health 99, 101–2
   and oral health 90
   and psoriasis 54
   and respiratory problems 76, 88

antibacterial properties 10, 26, 83,
   122, 139, 150

antifungal properties 26, 83

antigens 21

antihistamines, natural 76

antioxidants 15, 17, 18–22
   and age-related problems 51,
      69–71, 73–5
   and chronic problems 97, 104,
      97
   and gallstones 60
   and general infections 83
   and oral health 90
   and piles 101
   and respiratory problems 76–7
   and the skin 51, 79, 117
   see also specific antioxidants

antiseptic properties 78, 91
antiviral properties 26, 83
anxiety 67
apolipoprotein B 109
apoptosis (cell death) 18, 97, 98
arachidonic acid 74
arteries 107, 108, 110
arthritis 69, 70, 71
ascorbic acid 23
    see also vitamin C
asthma 76–7
astringents 117
atheroma 108, 110
atherosclerosis 107
athlete's foot 80

bacteria 28, 43, 51, 63, 116, 150
    see also antibacterial properties
banana treatment, rejuvenating 125
barbecue cleaner 143
barley, lemon barley water 34
baths
    circulation-boosting 66
    essential oils vapour 86
    exfoliating bath salts 123
beauty treatments 114–32
benefits of lemons 14–36
beta carotene (pro-vitamin A) 15,
    22
beta cryptoxanthin 22
betaglucuronidase 25, 88, 89
BHA (butylated hydroxyanisole) 26
BHT (butylated hydroxytoluene) 26
bifidobacteria 58, 84
bile, acidic 59
bins 141
bites 78
bitterness 41
black-rot fungus (Alternaria) 9
blackheads 117, 128
bleaching properties 131–2, 151
blood clots 110

blood flow 20, 22
blood pressure 20
    high 19, 97, 107, 108, 109, 110
blood sugar levels 97
    regulation 62, 64, 70, 98, 104–5
blood vessels 20, 44, 69, 78, 88,
    107, 110, 117
blood–brain barrier 20, 75
bone density 20
bowel cancer 18, 23, 24, 28, 98
bowel inflammation 24, 59
brain 74–5, 107, 110–11
breast cancer 23–25, 28, 98
bronchitis 88
browning, prevention 35
bruises 78
butylated hydroxyanisole (BHA) 26
butylated hydroxytoluene (BHT) 26
butyric acid 17, 24, 58, 84, 97,
    97–8, 108–9, 111
buying lemons 8–11

C-reactive protein 97, 97, 107–108,
    110–11
calcium 16, 23
    absorption 17, 64, 73, 74
    and ageing 69
    extraction from teeth/bones 62,
        69, 73
    and gallstones 59
    and heart disease 107
    and kidney stones 62
    and stress 67
calluses 44–7
cancer 18–21, 23–5, 28, 63, 69, 70,
    97–9
capillaries 20, 44, 88, 117
carcinogens 28, 29
carnitine 64
carotenoids 16, 18, 22, 54
carpet freshener 142
casein 10

cataracts 70
catarrh 83
cellulite 65
cellulose 16, 17, 58
ceviche 30
chamomile oil 56
chelation 21, 131
chemicals ix, 137, 138
chilblains 44
chlorophyll 22
cholesterol 17, 18, 20, 59
    HDL 17, 24, 97, 108–9, 111
    high 108–9
    LDL 20, 22–24, 107–11
chopping board rinse 150
chronic/serious conditions 104–11
cinnamon 84
circulation issues 26, 65–6
citral (lemonal) 25–6, 28–9, 129
citric acid 23–4, 54, 59, 116–7,
    131, 139, 150
citron trees x
Citrus 5
    C. maxima 5
    C. medica 5
    C. reticulate 5
citrus reamers 44
citrus trees x
citrus trumpets 45
citrus zesters 44
cleaning products, natural xii, 24,
    27, 45, 136–54
coconut oil 56
cold sores 81–2
cold-pressing 26
collagen 65, 79, 107
colon 58
colon cancer 18, 23–25, 28, 98
colour of lemons 8, 9, 10, 20,
    22–23
constipation 17, 58, 101
contraception 90

cooking with lemons 29–36
copper 16, 148
corns 44–6
coronary artery disease 107
coughs and colds 83–88
    soothing cough mixture 85
coumarins 18–19, 21–2, 25–6, 98,
    129
cuts 78
cypress oil 66, 103

dandruff 55–6
decongestants 83–4
deodorizing properties xii, 115, 122,
    141, 146
Department of Agriculture Pesticide
    Data Program 11
depression 67
dermatitis (skin inflammation) 21,
    116
descalers 144
diabetes 59, 69, 97, 104–95 107,
    110
    see also pre-diabetes
diarrhoea 17, 58–9
diet, healthy 29–30, 44
digestive aids 23, 49, 57, 60–5, 104
digestive problems 57–72
dipentene 27
diphenyl 11
disinfectant properties 150
distillation 26
diuretics 65
DNA (deoxyribonucleic acid)
    damage 19, 20
    mutation 97
docosahexaenoic acid 74
dysentery 43

E numbers 24
eczema 116
effervescents 24

eggs 35
elbows 128
energy content of lemons 16
Escherichia coli 58
ethyl alcohol 10
eucalyptus oil 86
Eureka lemon 6
evening primrose oil 120
exfoliating properties 24, 116, 117
    exfoliating bath salts 123
eye health 19, 22, 70–1

face masks
    anti-ageing 124
    brightening turmeric 126
    rejuvenating banana 125
fainting 98
`fast oxidizers' 98
fatigue 98–3
fats
    content of lemons 16
    digestion 60
    emulsification 60
    oxidation 18, 22
    triglyceride 64, 97, 107–9
    see also cholesterol; lipids
fever 83, 84
fibre xi, 16–18, 62, 88, 97, 108
fibroids 88
fingertip splits 128
first aid 78–7
fish 30, 36, 42, 50
flavonoids 18–22, 25, 41, 44
    and bronchitis 88
    and chronic illness 104, 98–108,
        110
    and first aid 78
    and piles 101
    and the skin 44, 54, 117
    and women's health 89
    see also hesperidin; rutin
flavourings 24

floor cleaner 144–5
flu 83–88
fluid retention 65
folic acid 94
food allergies/intolerances 50, 61–2
foot treatments 45
fractures 79
fragrance of lemons 129–30
free radicals 18, 73, 97, 107–9
fridges 141
fruit
    browning prevention 35
    production 5
fungi 9, 80, 116
    see also antifungal properties
fungicides 10, 11
furniture polish 149

gallbladder 59–60
    flush 60
gallstones 19, 59–60
ginger
    ginger oil 100
    honey, lemon and ginger tea 87
gingivitis 90
glucaric acid 23, 24–5, 89, 98, 110
glucuronidation 25, 28, 29, 89
glycaemic index 64, 104–9
grapefruit (*Citrus paradisi*) 5
graters 43
grazes 78
grease removal 143
grout whitener 143
growing lemons 4–8
gut bacteria 17
    and anaemia 57
    and chronic conditions 97,
        107–9, 111
    and diarrhoea 58
    and fibroids 88
    and immunity 84, 97
    and osteoporosis 73

gut health 57–64
hair care xii, 115, 131–2
    acidity of hair 117–18
    coloured hair 131
    DIY highlights xii, 132
    dry hair 131
    greasy hair 131
    hair problems 55–7
    lemon hair rinses 118
harvesting lemons 5
hay fever 76
HDL cholesterol 17, 24, 97, 108–9,
    111
head lice 57
headache 94
heart attack 19, 107, 109
heart disease 20, 22, 65, 69–70, 97,
    107–8
heartburn 60–1
heavy metals 21, 70, 131
Helicobacter pyrlori 63
herbicides 11
herby lemon steam cleanser 120
hesperidin 20, 59, 71, 75, 83, 101
homocysteine 74, 107, 110
humidifiers 141
hydrocarbons 25

IBS *see* irritable bowel syndrome
immunity 28, 84, 97
indigestion 28, 60–1
infections 19, 20, 22, 78–83
inflammation 63
    and age-related conditions 71,
        73–4
    and asthma 76
    bowel 24, 59
    and chronic conditions 107–8
    markers of 97, 97
    and metabolic syndrome 97
    see also anti-inflammatories
inflammatory bowel disease 24

inflammatory polyarthritis 71
inhalations 94
insect infestations 156
insecticides 10, 156
insomnia 95–6
insulin levels 62
invisible ink xii
iron 16, 57, 69
irritable bowel syndrome (IBS) 61
isomers 28
itching 54

joints 69, 71
juice x, 17, 35
    and the acid–alkaline balance
        69–70
    acidity 23, 24
    antioxidant content 19
    bottled xii, 45, 139
    buying lemons for 9
    dilution 50
    freezing 9
    how to take 50
    and invisible ink xii
    and natural beauty treatments
        55, 116–17, 121–7, 124–8,
        131–2
    and natural cleaning products
        139, 141, 143–4, 147–54
    and natural remedies 51–2,
        54–5, 58–65, 67, 70–1, 73–
        81, 87–92, 94, 97–9, 101–3,
        104–5, 108, 110–11, 128
    nutrients 16, 19, 23, 24
    preparation xi, 44–5
    storage 9

key lime (*Citrus aurantifolia*) 5
kidney problems 65
    kidney stones 62–3
kitchen deodorizers 141, 146

lactic acid 69–70
lactobacilli 58, 84
laundry 24, 25, 151–3
lavender oil 103, 128, 142, 145
LDL cholesterol 20, 22–4, 107–11
lemon barley water 34
lemon lore 35–6
lemon oil 16–17, 21–2, 25–9
    and anti-inflammatory massage
        oil 103
    and circulation-boosting baths
        66
    cold-pressing 26
    constituents 25–9
    and natural beauty treatments
        115, 118, 123
    and natural cleaning products
        140–47, 150, 156
    and natural remedies 47–111,
        67–8, 80–4, 86, 91–3, 95–7,
        99–101, 128
    soothing lemon oil 72
    storage 27
lemon slices 10, 35, 42–3, 50, 144
lemon squeezers 45
lemon tea 34
lemon tree (*Citrus limon*) x–xi, 5–8
lemon twists 43
lemon wedges 10, 42
lemon-producing countries 6
lemonade 83, 84
    classic 32
    variation 33
lettuce 36
leukaemia 98
lichenoid lesions 22
life expectancy 70
lime x
limescale 143, 144, 152
limonene 18, 25–8, 41
    and lemon fragrance 129
    and natural cleaning products
        147, 150, 156
    and natural remedies 61, 81,
        83, 89
limonin 16–18, 23, 41, 109
limonoids 18, 23, 98
linseed 85
lipids 115–16
lips, chapped 51
Lisbon lemon 6
liver 18, 25, 28–9, 89, 109–10
liver cancer 28
lung cancer 23, 28, 98

macular degeneration 71
magnesium 16, 62, 67, 73, 108
Malassezia furfur 55
mandarin 5, 6
manganese 16
massage oils 115, 128
    anti-inflammatory 103
    relaxing bedtime 96
    soothing 72
maximum permitted levels (MPL)
    11
memory loss 19, 73
mental health 67–8
metabolic syndrome 97
metal polishes 147–8
metals, heavy 21, 70, 131
Meyer `lemon' 6
microwave deodorizer 146
mildew 152
minerals 16, 17, 23, 89
mint 120
moisturizers xii, 24, 115–17, 119,
    122
mood lifters 140
moth repellents 156
mouth cancer 23, 98
mouth ulcers 92–3
mouthwash, antiseptic and astrin-
    gent 91

MPL *see* maximum permitted levels
muscle stiffness 99–100
myrrh oil 93

naringenin 20, 98
naringin 20, 41
natural remedies for health ix, xii,
    48–111
    age-related conditions 69–75
    allergies 76–7
    anaemia 57–8
    chronic/serious conditions
        104–11
    circulation issues 65–6
    coughs and colds 83–8
    digestive problems 57–64
    first aid 78–63
    general health 94–103
    hair conditions 55–7
    infections 78–63
    mental health 67–8
    oral health 90–3
    respiratory problems 76–7
    skin conditions 50–5
    women's health 88–90
neuralgia 101
nobiletin 20, 73, 99, 98
nutrients of lemons 15–25
nutritional supplements 18–19

obesity 59, 64, 97, 110
oestrogen 24–5, 51, 88–9
oils
    essential 26, 28, 56, 72, 86, 93,
        100, 103, 128, 138, 142, 145
    olive 149
    vitamin E 124
oral health 90–3
orange oil 26, 28
organic produce 9, 11
osteoporosis 69, 73–8
ovarian cancer 24–3

oxidation 18, 20, 22, 27, 35, 73–5,
    97, 107, 109–10, 117

pain 63, 101
panic attacks 67
parsley 120
pectin 17, 18
    and age-related conditions 73
    and chronic conditions 97–109,
        111
    and coughs and colds 84, 88
    and digestive problems 57–9,
        61, 64
    and heavy metal elimination 70
    and immunity 97
pedicures 127
peptic ulcer 63–4
periods, heavy 89
Persian lime (*Citrus latifolia*) 5
pesticides 7–8, 10, 11, 41
pH 62, 67, 69–70, 107
    blood 73, 94
    juice 23, 59, 139
    skin 115
    soap 116
    stomach 57, 59, 98, 104
    urine 67, 73, 80
phenolic compounds 16, 18–19,
    21–22, 44, 109
phosphorus 16
photosensitivity 21–22, 118
pigments 15, 22
pine oil 72
pips xi, 16–17, 23, 25
pith
    and buying lemons 9
    definition 16
    extraction xi
    and limonin 23
    and natural remedies 70, 71, 78
    nutrient content 16–19, 70
    and zesting 44

polishes 147–9
polymethoxylated flavones (PMFs) 20
polyphenols 19
 see also phenolic compounds
pomanders 140
pot pourri 140
potassium 16, 67, 108
potassium carbonate 61, 71
pre-diabetes 62, 97, 104, 108
prebiotics 58, 84, 98
preparing lemons 41–5
preservatives 10, 24, 26, 35, 45
preserved lemons 31
probiotics 58, 84
progesterone 88–9
prostate cancer 24–5, 28, 98
protein 16, 60–2, 77, 98
psoralens 21–2, 54
psoriasis 54–5

quercetin 20–1, 75–6, 83, 88, 98
 see also rutin

respiratory problems 76–7
restlessness 101–2
rheumatoid arthritis 71
ripening lemons 22
room spritzers 140
rutin 21, 65, 78, 101, 117, 128
 see also quercetin

salicylic-acid salts 17
salt 123, 143, 152
satiety 64
scalps 56, 117–18
scent of lemons 129–30
sebum 50, 116, 117
sedative properties 20, 95, 101
selenium 16, 18, 62, 94
shampoo 24, 117, 131
Shigella 43

short-chain fatty acids 17, 57–58, 73, 84, 97, 97, 107–109, 111
shower cleaner 152
skin
 acidity 115–16
 ageing 19, 51, 69
 hard 128
 photosensitivity 21–2
skin cancer 23, 98
skin conditions 21–3, 22, 50–5, 98, 128
skincare 115–16
 cleansers xii, 115–16, 119–20
 daily routines 119–22
 face masks 124–6
 moisturizers xii, 24, 115–17, 119, 122
 toners 119, 121
soaps 10, 24–5, 116, 131
sodium 57, 62–4, 74, 77, 98–9, 104
sodium metabisulfite 45
sour properties x, 23
spa treatments, home 122–7
sprains 79
stain removal 151–3
staphylococci 43
statins 109
stings 78
stomach acid 28
 deficiency 23, 57–64, 69, 74, 76–7, 98–9, 104
 pH level 57, 59, 98, 104
stomach cancer 23, 28, 98, 107
storing lemons 9–11, 35
stress 67–8, 107
stroke 19, 70, 97, 107, 109–11
sunburn 19, 21, 79–80
super-flavonoids 20
surface cleaners 143, 150, 152
sweat patch removal 151
sweet almond oil 45, 72, 80, 82, 93, 100–1, 103, 118, 128

tangeretin 20, 98
taste of lemons 41
tea
    black 98
    honey, lemon and ginger 87
    lemon 34
tea tree oil 86, 93, 145
terpenes 25–8, 129
    see also limonene
terpenoids 23, 28
toxins, elimination 18, 29
triglyceride fats 64, 97, 107–9
turmeric mask, brightening 126

ulcer, peptic 63–4
uric acid 62
urine
    pH 67, 73, 80
    production 65
urine infections 80

vegetables, browning prevention 35
veins 65, 101
    broken 117, 128
    varicose 102
vetivert oil 96
vinegar 70, 94, 104–5, 138, 144–6
vitamin A 22
vitamin B 15, 62, 67, 88, 94, 98
    deficiency 69, 74
vitamin C (ascorbic acid) xi, 15,
    17–19, 23
    and age-related problems 70,
        71, 73
    and chronic illness 104, 109
    and collagen 65, 79
    and coughs and colds 83
    deficiency 69
    and fibroids 88
    and flavonoids 20
    and hot water and lemon 49
    and immunity 97

and infertility 94
and piles 101
and the skin 117
and stress 67
supplements 19
and weight loss 64
vitamin E 15, 18, 94, 124

wardrobe fresheners 140
warts 54
washing lemons 11, 41
washing up boosters 144
water cleanser 150
water intake 83
water retention 24
water-softeners 24
waxed lemons 10–11, 41
weight loss 64, 108
white blood cells 28, 97, 107
window cleaner 143

ylang ylang oil 96, 128

zest 16, 35
    and age-related problems 70–1,
        73–5
    and chronic illness 104–5, 108,
        110–11
    and circulation issues 65, 128
    and coughs and colds 88
    and digestive problems 58–61,
        63–4
    and first aid 78–9
    and general health 94, 97–9,
        101–2
    and mental health 67
    preparation xi, 9, 43–4
    and skin conditions 44, 55
    and women's health 88–9
    zesty sugar 44
zinc 16, 18, 67, 73, 94